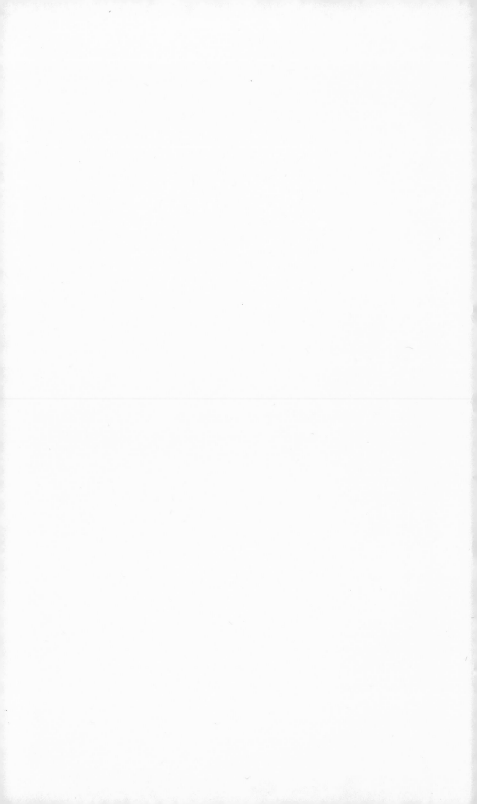

THE MAKING OF A WOMAN VET

OF A

WOMAN VET

Sally Haddock, D.V.M.

with Kathy Matthews

SIMON AND SCHUSTER NEW YORK

Copyright © 1985 by Sally Haddock and Kathy Matthews

All rights reserved including the right of reproduction in whole or in
part in any form

Published by Simon and Schuster,
A Division of Simon & Schuster, Inc.
Simon & Schuster Building
Rockefeller Center
1230 Avenue of the Americas
New York, New York 10020

SIMON AND SCHUSTER and colophon are registered trademarks
of Simon & Schuster, Inc.

Designed by Jennie R. Nichols/Levavi & Levavi

Manufactured in the United States of America

1   3   5   7   9   10   8   6   4   2

Library of Congress Cataloging in Publication Data

Haddock, Sally.
The making of a woman vet.

1. Haddock, Sally.   2. Veterinarians—New York (N.Y.)
—Biography.   3. Women veterinarians—New York (N.Y.)—
Biography.   I. Matthews, Kathy, date.   II. Title.
SF613.H27A34   1985   636.089'092'4 [B]   85-10778

ISBN 0-671-49967-X

ACKNOWLEDGMENTS

People and pets too numerous to mention have helped in the preparation of this book, but I would like to take the opportunity to thank just a few. I am particularly grateful to:

My wonderful parents for all their love, support and encouragement through all my years.

Dr. Ralph E. Headley of Oxford, Ohio, for being so compassionate and for giving me that first veterinary job that meant so much.

My friends for their patience and enthusiasm, especially Dr. Lorraine Harper, Nancy "Skid" Skidmore, Shelley Schalip, Dr. Lesley Smith and Dr. Donna Stafford, and also to Becky Wilcox Oltean, who unknowingly inspired me to become a veterinarian.

Dr. Patrick Bredel and Dr. Sue Harris of Pittsburgh, Pennsylvania, for giving me confidence during my first year as a veterinarian.

Dr. William Kay, Director of the Animal Medical Center, and his staff for a unique opportunity to spend three years learning more than I could have learned anywhere else.

5

Dr. Dennis Zawie and Dr. Michael Garvey, the gastroenterologists of the Animal Medical Center, for their patience and invaluable guidance in the specialized training of endoscopy.

Dr. Paul Kaplan of New York City for being an outstanding veterinarian as well as a great friend.

My husband, Tom, for his unfailing love, support and understanding as well as his unending love for animals.

Tommy and Jason for their continual support and cooperation.

The staff of Veselka Coffee Shop for providing Kathy and me with countless delicious breakfasts and a place to meet.

My pets for their constant inspiration and affection: Tajma and Noir, my cats; Claus and Frito, my birds; and especially Myriah, my lovable golden retriever— the world's greatest jogging partner.

My very special patients who keep me enthusiastic about my work and who reward me in so many ways, especially Dolly, the French Bulldog; Bunny Celeste; Cinder and Boogie, the cats; Phillip, the English Cocker; Rocky, the poddle; and Mabel, the yellow-naped Amazon parrot.

John Boswell, whose twenty-three-year-old cat, Marie, first brought us together and who encouraged me to write this book.

And Patricia Soliman, whose love for animals and editorial skills contributed enormously to this book.

To my husband
Tom
for whom words
cannot express my love

CONTENTS

PROLOGUE: THE RESURRECTION OF BUNNY CELESTE

Miracles are one of the fringe benefits of veterinary medicine. Bunny Celeste was my first genuine miracle.

Bunny Celeste came to us at the Animal Medical Center, a vision in pink and black, in the early morning hours of the worst blizzard of the winter of 1982–83. The "Blizzard of '83," as the press dubbed it before you could even make a footprint in the snow, eventually surpassed every weatherperson's dreams. For seventy-two hours there was no news but snow news.

I was on a double shift and that Friday night was the quietest I'd ever spent at the AMC. As I'd made my way the following morning from the subway station to the center, I heard the sound of a muffled horn honking nearby on Second Avenue. As the streets had not been plowed and there was absolutely no traffic, I'd wondered who it could be. As the honking approached I saw that it was a newspaper delivery truck. Before each store a bundle of newspapers flew from the truck into a snowdrift somewhere near the store entrance. The driver must have been honking to let the owners know the papers had arrived; they were all quickly buried by the falling snow.

The city was blanketed with twenty-four inches of snow. Most of the people who lived in New Jersey or on Long Island had been unable to make it in and we were huddled like cheerful survivors in the AMC lounge trading BD/LD stories. BD/LD stories are the tragic accounts of big dog/little dog encounters that send the participants to a veterinary emergency room. The odds are usually in the big dog's favor, but the outcome can depend more on personality and breed than size. A twenty-four-inch bull terrier can readily best a forty-three-inch Irish wolfhound. The real issue of BD/LD encounters is not who wins the fight, but what can be salvaged of the survivors.

One common problem with a BD/LD, aside from loss of dignity and a shocking amount of noise, is puncture wounds. Even though a puncture can appear to be nothing more than a tiny hole, the tissue beneath the skin is ripped often, and you must cut open the surrounding flesh in order to thoroughly clean out the bacteria, hair or dirt beneath the skin. The procedure is about as messy as the original fight and, if it was a championship bout, you can spend a long time putting things to rights. A dog in with a few small puncture wounds can wind up looking like a patchwork puppy.

Normally BD/LD victims reach us after the fight, but one night there was an encounter right in our waiting area. When the dust cleared it proved one of the most tragic BD/LD's ever. A mastiff was waiting at our sign-in desk with his owner. It was Westminster Dog Show time and the mastiff was in town for the competition. Suddenly, while being groomed at the show, the dog had snapped at his handler. The handler didn't know if the dog was ill or simply irritated by the commotion that reigns as thousands of dogs prepare to meet their moment of reckoning.

When a mastiff snaps, attention must be paid. The ancient Romans used to toss fighting mastiffs into the amphitheaters when they ran out of Christians and lions. It's not just their personalities, it's their size. As an eighteenth-century mastiff fancier once said, "As a lion is to a cat, so is the mastiff to a dog." In the past few hundred decades, I'm happy to report, the breed has shown a far greater improvement in temperament than their owners can boast, and today they're prized as companions as well as bodyguards and watch dogs. I've known some extraordinarily sweet and gentle mastiffs. But, at an average of 180 pounds, they are still formidable.

This particular mastiff was sitting calmly in the lobby of the AMC until another dog, a German shepherd, was led into his ken. A classic BD/LD ensued and in the midst of the truly terrifying melee, the owner of the mastiff was bitten in the leg by his own dog. Nearly the entire calf muscle was removed by the mastiff's jaws. The man was a diabetic and this caused complications. Ultimately, his leg had to be amputated.

The mastiff was left at the AMC for weeks while his fate was being decided elsewhere. He was locked in a cage with a combination lock. This was the only time I've ever seen a dog locked in a cage at the AMC. He was fed through the bars and soiled newspaper was pulled from beneath the cage and replaced with fresh. We observed him for signs of rabies and eventually grew fond of him. He seemed calm and friendly enough, though certainly no one trusted him. Eventually he was put to sleep. The final cost in both money and pain of that BD/LD encounter was the highest I've encountered.

By the time we ran out of BD/LD stories, it was 10 A.M. Saturday. Not a single case had turned up the previous night. A new record for the Animal Medical Center. We had been sitting around for an hour now without a single case. When my name was called over the paging system, everyone laughed, certain it was a joke.

The reason for my summons turned out to be Bunny Celeste. Bunny Celeste was a three-year-old black rabbit with all the optimistic dignity that makes rabbits such good companions. As the snowflakes melted into her fine glossy coat, she observed me with one clear eye and one blinking one. Her mistress had carried her, swaddled in towels, all the way across

Central Park from the Upper West Side. In a scene that must have resembled a trans-Siberian trek, Bunny Celeste & Co. had probably been the only creatures thus far to successfully cross the snowbound city.

Celeste, her mistress explained, had been on a decline. Her eye was running and she was listless. What was most alarming was that she hadn't eaten a morsel of food in three days. Snowstorm or not, Celeste needed attention.

Bunny Celeste was clearly the apple of her mistress's eye, and the poor woman seemed to be shouldering more than half of Celeste's distress. It's common for a pet owner to suffer more visibly than the animal in the teeth of a malady. The uncomplaining stoicism of most pets is what can be so heart-breaking to their owners. And I can't help but be affected by the unhappiness of any pet owner who comes to me. I try to keep my emotions in check, but when I encounter a sick animal and a desperately worried loving owner and I'm an ice cube on a tar roof in July. Also, because of Watson, a memorable rabbit from vet school days, I have a special feeling for the species so I was bound and determined to get Celeste back in shape as soon as possible.

I examined Celeste and saw that she had an upper respiratory infection called "snuffles." Snuffles, a common disease of rabbits, is caused by an invading bacteria. It produces sneezing and runny eyes. Once a rabbit's nose is running it can't smell, and when it can't smell it loses all interest in eating. If caught in the early stages, snuffles usually responds quickly to antibiotics so I explained the situation to Celeste's mistress and gave her medication, instructions and encouragement. She was obviously relieved just to have something to do that would help her pet.

Because things were so quiet, and to get a look at the storm, I walked Celeste and her mistress down the ramp to the exit of the AMC. It was still snowing but at least you could see across Sixty-second Street to the other side. The drifts were something else altogether. It looked like giant clouds of snow had fallen intact to the pavement. I'd never seen anything like it in the city. It was still and majestic and beautiful. But of course all I had to do was climb the ramp to the next floor; Celeste and her mistress were headed back across nearly thirty blocks of snow mountains. I felt like someone waving good-bye to a pioneer as she strapped the piano to the buckboard to head into the unknown.

Two days later, when the snowdrifts had turned gray and oceans of slush surged at the curbsides, Celeste again appeared at the AMC. As she described Celeste's symptoms, her mistress's hands never left her rabbit, who was lying patiently on the examining table. Her attachment to Celeste was intense. She was an artist who spent much of her time alone in her studio with only Celeste for company, muse and encouragement. She was frantic with worry.

Celeste still would eat nothing. Her mistress, on my instructions, was trying to force-feed her gruel a few times a day but Celeste was resisting. She was also giving Celeste antibiotic injections.

The most difficult aspect of the situation was that the more her owner worked to make her well, the more Celeste grew to distrust and fear her. Where previously Celeste had greeted her mistress with enthusiasm and often approached her to be cuddled, now she hid at the sight of her. In Celeste's eyes her mistress had been transformed from an unqualified source of care and affection to a virtual torturer. Her efforts to force-feed Celeste and to give her injections were upsetting both of them almost as much as the actual illness. It was as if they had both lost their best friends.

I was pleased to discover after examining her that Celeste's snuffles were clearing up, but I knew I had to find a way to make her eat. Her mistress's condition as much as Celeste's demanded that I find the problem and correct it.

I found myself, as I so often do, wishing that Celeste could speak up. I wanted Walt Disney. No more of this mute cuteness; I wanted an earful of specific complaints like "It hurts when I hop. I have a headache and my cage is in a dreadful draft. And you might want to know that I've been eating lead-paint chips." It's one of the frustrations and challenges of veterinary medicine. The patient can't speak, can't give you the crucial information you need. It's often, to some degree, a matter of guesswork.

I decided to file Celeste's molars. Rabbits' top and bottom molars do not meet exactly. The areas that overlap do not get ground down by everyday chewing and over time may form points on the overlapped edges. These points pinch the cheek when chewing and can cause much pain to the rabbit. If this happens to a healthy rabbit, it will pick food up in its mouth and then just drop it; the pain of chewing is too great. Naturally, this condition will affect the rabbit's appetite.

Celeste didn't seem to be interested in food at all—she wasn't even sniffing the tidbits she was offered—but I thought that filing her teeth would be worth a try. I sedated her and filed her teeth down to a more reasonable bunny-like size and gave her fluids subcutaneously to help replenish her nutrition and prevent dehydration. I prescribed Nutrical—a nourishing caloric supplement that comes in a sort of toothpaste tube. A few dabs of Nutrical, if her mistress could convince her to take them, would give Celeste strength. She certainly couldn't go on forever without food. I sent them off and hoped for the best.

When Celeste's mistress called a few days later, my heart sank. She reported that Celeste was lying on her side on the floor of her cage, her little paws drawn in tight to her body. She still wouldn't eat and now was utterly terrified of her mistress. She would run and hide at the sound of her footsteps or her key in the lock. Celeste was becoming the invisible rabbit and it looked like she'd decided, as she'd lost everything that made her life worth living, she was simply going to die.

The situation was unbearable. Celeste's mistress couldn't bear to watch her suffer. She couldn't bear to fill Celeste's last days with injections and force-feeding and pain. Most of all, she couldn't bear to lose the love of her bunny, who'd grown so frightened of her that her very presence made Celeste anxious. She had no hope. She was bringing Celeste into the AMC to be put to sleep.

When Bunny Celeste, her mistress and I met in the examining room, only Celeste was unmoved. She was slightly less active than usual and had lost some weight but still had her bright-eyed curiosity as she nosed about the floor of the room sniffing inquisitively. In fact, I was surprised to see Celeste looking so well. The trust that an animal has for its owner sometimes, especially at moments like these, seems a cruel joke. Even Celeste, nervous at the hands of her mistress, had no real fear. In fact, I began to think that this bunny, though obviously wan and weak, was not nearly so sick as her mistress believed. I didn't really want to give up on Celeste, but it seemed there was nothing to be done; animals were animals and people were people and this woman was being driven to desperation by the sickness of her companion. And I couldn't guarantee that Celeste would eventually be cured.

It's enormously difficult for a pet owner who loves his animal to make the decision to put it to sleep. After all, pets are in most cases beloved friends. But Celeste's mistress had seen her pet degenerate from a dear companion into an animal that cringed at her approach. She had no hope that Celeste would get well and had agonized over what direction to take. She'd reached her decision and I didn't feel that I could or should try to dissuade her.

I was fighting my tears but Celeste's mistress was weeping openly as she stroked her pet's fur for what would be the last time. Finally our miserable trio was broken up, and cradling Celeste's small body in my arms, I headed for one of the back wards. Unless an owner insisted on being present, it was better to put an animal to sleep out of sight. Oftentimes once they're injected with the drug they have involuntary muscular contractions. It's upsetting enough to have a pet put to sleep; it's usually unbearable to watch twitches and grimaces.

As Bunny Celeste crouched on the stainless-steel table, her nose twitched occasionally but she was otherwise still and solemn. I held the bottle of euthanasia solution and watched Celeste.

And I couldn't do it. I didn't really believe that Celeste was as sick as her mistress thought. I thought Bunny Celeste deserved more of a chance. Most animal owners will want to fight for their pets long after the trained eye of the vet knows the case is hopeless. But with Bunny Celeste I believed that the psychological trauma of watching her rabbit suffer gradually eroded her mistress's hope. She simply loved Bunny Celeste too much.

I held Celeste on the table and decided to take a risk. I'd give her a few more days of life and do everything I could to make her well. If there was no improvement I'd honor her mistress's wishes. But I didn't even want to think about that; I just wanted Celeste well and home again.

I lifted Celeste, nose twitching, ignorant of her brush with death. I carried her up two floors to a quiet ward where I knew she'd be unnoticed. I gave her an injection of fluids to help with her dehydration. I administered some antibiotics. Everything I did seemed like an apology. Finally I made her as comfortable as I could in an out-of-the-way cage. I put my palm on her chest before I left her. There was that fast small-animal heartbeat.

Bunny Celeste hovered like a sky jumper at the plane door for another three days. Her snuffles seemed to be clearing up, but she still wouldn't eat. I was forcing fluids and nourishment. I was convinced she could get better; I just had to convince *her* of that.

On the fourth day of my Bunny Celeste vigil a package arrived for me at the reception desk. I opened it to discover a large chocolate bunny. Accompanying the bunny was a note written in beautiful calligraphy. It thanked me for all the time, care and sympathy I had given the late beloved Bunny Celeste. Her mistress was becoming reconciled to her loss, the note said, but it had taken a few days. She had wanted to write to me immediately after Celeste's death, but her sorrow was too great.

I was stunned. Now that the woman had overcome her grief, would it be fair to present her with a resurrected Celeste, even if I could? Would she be able to cope with the situation? What kind of mess had I gotten myself into?

Within another day, the Tuesday before Easter, in fact, Celeste began to eat. As the signs of snuffles had disappeared, I had taken her off antibiotics. Sometimes antibiotics can take away an animal's appetite and I wanted to see how she would do once they were discontinued. By that time a number of people at the AMC knew about Celeste, "the Secret Rabbit," and everyone was rooting for her.

By Holy Thursday, Celeste had made nearly a complete recovery. She was glossy and spirited and absolutely ravenous. The tender leaves of watercress I used to tempt her disappeared along with the ignoble rabbit pellets. Celeste was cured.

Now I had to deal with Celeste's future and it was a task I undertook with great reluctance. I made a few phone calls and hoped for the best.

I wasn't present at the resurrection of Bunny Celeste but the reports that drifted back to me after the event made me know I'd done the right thing.

Easter dawned cool and rainy in New York. It certainly wasn't weather to celebrate. Celeste's mistress was collecting herself for the day when her boyfriend rang from the lobby of her building. She buzzed him inside. When she heard his knock at the door, she called out that it was open. After a few seconds he hadn't come in so she went over to the door and opened it.

Her boyfriend held a large carton that advertised a 1982 Beaujolais. "Happy Easter," he said as he handed the carton to her.

She must have been surprised that she could so easily hold a case of wine. But her greater surprise came when one flap of the carton pushed open and a familiar black bunny greeted her. At first she couldn't believe her eyes. She lifted Celeste from the carton and cradled her against her chest. Celeste, well and happy, was delighted to be home.

It was a joyous reunion and perhaps Bunny Celeste's happiest Easter.

And looking back to my first glimmering of a hope that one day I'd be a vet, it seemed almost a miracle that it had ever happened.

THE FIRST HILL

The difference between riding in a car and riding on a bike is hills. I had been along this road in Oxford, Ohio, countless times. It meandered its way past the university stables, past the fields and silos, past the cows and little old houses with green shutters. But I'd always thought of it as flat. Now, hills were humping up at a truly alarming rate. For every fence post, tree and heifer there was a corresponding hill. On top of the hills there were rocks, ruts, branches, half a state's worth of dust and now and again a cow pie. As omens go, I thought, this ride is a bad one.

There was a lot at stake. It was beginning to seem that my whole future was hanging on that ride. I was on my way to ask for a job. It was one of those simple events in life that nonetheless would be a turning point for me and I knew it. There I was panting along like "The Little Engine That Could," knowing this job would be the beginning or the end of my career, and the road was getting longer and the hills higher.

It was autumn, a crisp bright day that made you think of football games and sports cars. I had a week before the first quarter of my senior year at Miami University. When you mention Miami University, most people say things like "Surfing major?" or "You must be pale because you're always partying." In fact, Miami University is about as far as you can get from Florida and riotous living. It's in the lower left-hand corner of Ohio. It's a relentlessly academic state school. It's in farm country and hasn't seen a wave suitable for any kind of sport since the glacier receded billions of years ago. We had our fun, of course, but it's no party school.

At the same time I suppose it's fair to wonder why, if they're so smart at Miami U., they haven't come up with a more accurate name for themselves. Fortunately Miami University is located in the town of Oxford. This is redeeming as one can always respond to the question "Where did you go to school?" with the literal and impressive geographic answer.

So there I was back in Oxford again for my senior year and I'd decided once and for all that I wanted to become a veterinarian after having toyed with the idea on many occasions. I'd worked my way through all the usual career way stations. I'd majored in psychology for a short time but I found it a frustrating discipline because it seemed to me to hold more questions than answers. So I switched to zoology. Then I began to dally with the teaching profession. Even though I was a zoology major, teaching seemed to offer a more concrete way to meet the financial demands of adult life. There certainly wasn't a lot of call for zoologists that I knew of. My parents and most everybody else thought teaching was a fine idea.

I'll admit that my interest in teaching wasn't entirely practical: I'd designed a glamorous apprenticeship for myself. Did you know that you can student-teach abroad? Or at least once upon a time you could. Or maybe someone was pulling my leg right from the outset. No matter. My head teemed with visions of me sipping cappuccino in Florence, exploring ruins and tacos in Mexico City and so on. Though teaching was a practical and, given my international plan, exciting exit out of the career question, I never pictured myself coming to grips in a hands-on fashion with the actual imparting of knowledge to small, eager minds. So when the student-teaching-abroad dream dissolved, the lure of chalk and lesson plans went with it.

The decision to become a vet didn't really come out of left field. In fact, it was more discovery than decision, and I suppose that's true of the best career choices. When all my other career notions were chipped away, what remained was an aspiring vet. I had dreamed about becoming a vet ever since childhood, but had always assumed it would be impossible for me to be accepted by a veterinary college.

It is not easy to become a veterinarian. But once I'd settled on it, I wanted to become one more than anything in the world. I truly loved animals, but it was more than that. I loved the intricacies of science. I liked knowing how a stray amoeba could wreak havoc with a digestive system. I liked understanding the delicate mechanism of life. Veterinary medicine offered the answers I missed in psychology. It was more practical than zoology. It was a "hands-on" science with a clear goal.

There were about twenty-two veterinary colleges in the United States when I was applying. A few new ones have been built very recently and they would up today's total. Still, even at twenty-five or twenty-eight, that's not a lot. For many people there's only one school they can apply to: the veterinary college in their state. Vet schools don't like out-of-state applicants; they have enough problems fitting in their own people. Of course some states have no vet school at all and they make arrangements with others to handle their aspiring students. If I wanted to be a vet, I had to be accepted at the Ohio State University College of Veterinary Medicine. One out of every ten applicants would be accepted.

In order to meet the unofficial requirements for admittance to a vet school, I desperately needed a job with a veterinarian. (Most of these jobs are voluntary.) Most veterinary colleges will not take a serious look at an application from a student who has not worked with animals. Many people imagine they would like to become vets but what they'd really like to be are dog trainers, zoo keepers, cat sitters or parakeet mavens, and vet schools don't want people to find this out on their time. They are bound and determined to impress on prospective candidates the less savory aspects of animal care. The blood and guts, the endless hours. An affection for animals, no matter how sincere and enduring, won't carry a student through the difficult science courses, the sometimes gruesome aspects of autopsies and surgeries, and the stern discipline that veterinary medicine demands.

Now one might guess that a bright, eager volunteer with serious ambitions would be embraced with enthusiasm by any established vet. But I had spent a good part of my summer scouting for one who would let me come and clean the kennels, hold down fierce animals or do anything that would demonstrate how determined I was about the profession. I'd presented myself to vet after vet and they'd looked at me as if I'd just asked to borrow their Buick and a few hundred dollars. Ohio seemed to be filled with vets who had a future-vet cousin or niece slaving away on the premises. I had no connections at all. It was difficult for me not to resent students who already had a connection in the field, though at the same time I desperately wished that I had one too.

I also didn't have a 4.0 grade average, which some of the rejecting vets whom I approached for a job found shocking. That summer more than one person told me to give up on the idea of veterinary school and try medical school instead.

The cheering section that had supported my teaching aspirations had deserted me when I'd decided on becoming a vet. In fact in my freshman year, when I'd first toyed with becoming a vet, I'd been so quickly discouraged by reports of how demanding and competitive vet school was that I'd lowered my sights immediately. I had announced that I'd transfer to the Animal Care Technology Program at the University of Cincinnati. This was a two-year program which would give me a career with animals and some connection with science. Though I wouldn't be a vet, at least I'd be working with animals and doing something that interested me.

I think I was inspired to make this decision by the architecture in the town of Oxford. In Oxford you won't find a building over three stories high. The reason for this, as I understand it, is that the firemen can't reach any higher. The lesson was as follows: assess your limitations and proceed accordingly. The Animal Care Technology Program was my "low-rise" alternative.

But my parents, as parents will, stepped in. As the Cincinnati program gave only a two-year degree, my parents thought it was like being a High Church Episcopalian instead of a Catholic—a half measure. If you're going to spend a lot of time and money in school, you might as well go whole hog and get a four-year degree. So I had briefly forgotten about vet school and moved on to other things. But that was my freshman year. Now I was almost a senior and had learned something: determination counts. I wasn't going to be easily discouraged this time. I was going to quit listening to everyone else and follow my heart.

That's how I found myself pumping away on that beautiful September morning, swallowing dust and trying to keep control of the hand brakes with crossed fingers. I'd passed the animal hospital that was my destination plenty of times, though I didn't really know anything about it. As I pumped away, I imagined a large sign at its gate: "Last Chance Animal Hospital."

When I finally rolled up the driveway I was disappointed to find a neat, well-tended clapboard building. It was clear I couldn't volunteer to pick weeds or paint shutters until I worked my way up to cage cleaner. The waiting room was small and neat. I joined the two other people there, both holding cats. If they thought it strange that I was visiting the vet without a pet they didn't reveal it.

When my name was called I strode into the examining room with borrowed confidence. The vet was young. Just a bit older than I and this cheered me. Perhaps he'd been through this desperate job hunt recently enough to be sympathetic. Maybe I'd have a chance. I waited for him to meet my eyes so I could introduce myself but he kept staring at my feet. Were my sneakers untied? Were my socks unmatched? Finally I realized he must be looking for a pet, a dog or cat that would explain my visit. I took a breath and launched into my introduction and plea.

"Sorry, we're all booked up, miss."

He still wouldn't meet my eyes. Then I knew. He'd no doubt already had brushes with desperate Miami University students. He probably found it easier to give out the bad news without ever looking into his applicants' eyes. I paused, willing him to look at me, to make me the exception. I felt sorry for him but I couldn't afford to make it easy.

"I'll do anything. Maybe fill in during the night. I could exercise the dogs. I've had a lot of zoology courses."

Still no eye contact.

"I can cook."

At least I got him to look up. I recognized his expression. It was that of a cornered animal.

Shaking his head, he said, "Try the town vet, miss. Good luck."

I didn't want to cry when I left his office in case there was anyone in the waiting room. They'd surely think my pet had died and maybe they'd say something to comfort me and then I'd really lose control. Besides, trying for this job was a long shot. Still, there was a lump in my throat and my eyes were stinging. The waiting room was empty and I closed the door quietly as I left.

The hills were even higher on the return trip, the dust thicker and the temptation to sink into a morass of self-pity overwhelming. This was what everyone had warned me about. Friends, teachers, veterinarians and even, it seemed, passers-by had told me that it was just too difficult, too competitive, too demanding. But I had really believed I could make a go of it. Now, pedaling along, I felt foolish. What vet school would take me if I didn't get a job? And there didn't seem to be a person other than myself in the state of Ohio who thought I was vet material.

Then I remembered that the young vet had mentioned the

vet in town. I recalled a small sign just the other side of the railroad tracks. As long as I'd virtually crossed the Alps by bike, another block or two wouldn't matter. It would give me something to focus on, a few more minutes of optimism. I'd give the town vet a try.

Passing through the town of Oxford is short work. There's a scattering of churches, a bookstore and a few bars which represent faith, hope and charity, in that order, to the students at Miami U. The vet's office was just outside of town. It was surrounded by a white picket fence. The office itself, really a converted garage, had an appealing down-at-the-heels air. But when I entered the waiting room I thought this, too, would be a futile effort. It was empty. No patients equals slow practice equals no job. I leaned back out the door to ring the bell and stood waiting, giving myself another minute, another two minutes, before I turned tail and ran.

The man who finally appeared in the doorway was brushing crumbs from the front of his white lab coat and I guessed that I was interrupting his lunch. There was a moment of awkwardness. How could I expect him to need help when he didn't have any patients? Before he even managed to collect himself and tell me to apply to medical school, I recited my brave spiel.

He wasn't watching my feet. He was peering at me intently through his bifocals as he continued brushing at invisible crumbs. Finally he offered me a hand to shake.

"Delighted to meet you, Miss Haddock. You say you'd like a job?"

Even this slender encouragement was like a drug to me.

"I'm a zoology major at Miami and I want to go to vet school. It could be volunteer, of course. Anytime that's convenient for you. But I can't skip classes ... well, most classes. ..."

He was still peering at me with great intensity.

Finally he broke the silence. "Perhaps you could lend a hand during the evening hours?"

Having just let go of his hand, I grabbed it again.

"Yes, wonderful. That'll be fine. That'll be great. When do I start?"

When at last he disengaged his hand he was smiling the warmest smile I'd ever seen. I had to blink hard to hide my tears.

As I picked my way across the railroad tracks on my return trip I saw the future rolling out like a broad meadow before me. I had a job with a vet. He seemed to be a very kind and decent vet, for that matter. Now all I had to do was work hard at it and learn all I could, study like a demon to boost my grade point average, sign up for every science course that would have me, be one of the 10 percent of all applicants who's admitted to veterinary college and, with more than a little luck, in five years I'd be a veterinarian.

FRESHMAN YEAR

FIRST DAYS

Ohio State University is a huge sprawl of buildings that seems to begin just as the city of Columbus peters out. Most of the campus is a random mix of high modern towers and low brick buildings that spread haphazardly until they cross the Olentangy River. To get to the vet school you leave the cluster of old ivy-covered buildings that form the heart of the school, drive along a street lined with more fast-food establishments than mind or stomach can encompass, past the great OSU stadium, past the first supermarket in the United States—a squat unprepossessing brick structure with an apron of parking lot—and finally you cross the river. Here the buildings for the School of Agriculture and the College of Veterinary Medicine are less crowded, more modern and there's an immediate feeling that the workings of the schools depend more on the outdoors than the insides of classrooms and libraries. I had visited the vet school before but arriving on my first official day as a student, filled with enthusiasm and high hopes, everything seemed fresh and vivid despite the Indian summer heat.

That first day seemed a thrilling beginning to a new life. There had been so many times in the past year that I thought it would never happen. To think that in four years I would leave the campus a vet at last would mean the realization of a dream. After the long hours of filling out forms, being inter-

29

viewed, filling out still more forms, getting my voluntary job with a vet, it was finally happening—I was a vet student.

I remembered my admission interview. It had been a last-minute business. I'd called OSU about the results of my application to see if I qualified for an interview; it was already way past the time when I should have heard from them. I learned that some applications had been lost or mislaid, mine among them. But the professor who gave me this news told me to come up for an interview anyhow. When? How about tomorrow? So I grabbed a ride with a friend and, a bundle of apprehension, I appeared the next morning. I thought the interview had gone badly—I just hadn't had answers for a few of the questions because I hadn't had enough experience. I had been honest and said I didn't know. By the time I left I thought that this time out I'd most likely be rejected. Still, I could reapply the following year. I wasn't totally demoralized. I could take more courses in the intervening year and better my chances of eventual acceptance.

While passing through Columbus after graduation from college I had stopped by the vet school to see what courses they would recommend for continuing education, courses that would help me when I reapplied to the vet school. I had by then decided that I certainly wouldn't be accepted the first time around. I had, after all, heard many stories of vet students only being accepted after their third, fourth and even fifth applications. When I at last found my way to the admissions office I explained my questions about continuing education courses to one of the vets there. "Are you sure you've been rejected?" he asked. When I said that I wasn't, he called to his secretary, "Is Sally Haddock in the 'dead file'?" The dead file! Well, I wasn't there and so there was still a shred of hope.

And then in the summer I received an envelope from the vet school and it was a thick envelope, not the one-page letter of condolence and rejection I'd been expecting. And now, despite all the false starts, here I was, gazing in awe at upper-class vet students in white coats who looked so quintessentially professional with their instruments in their pockets. Everything impressed me, from the inside of the labs to the giant coolers. As I moved my things into my room, I resolved to work and study as hard as I could so that when I finally got out into practice, I would be the best vet possible, a vet I would have been happy to bring my *own* dog to.

On that first day of vet school we got small hints of the strange world we were entering and how profoundly it would change us. It began with language. We were all given a booklet filled with basic vet school information. At the bottom of one page, in a little box, was a collection of letters most of us wound up reading that first night. Under the heading "Abbreviations You Might Find Useful" it listed: CBC—Complete Blood Count; WBC—White Blood Count; RBC—Red Blood Count; and finally, the mysterious HBC—Hit by Car. Could this be part of a bizarre hazing ritual in which they lined us up, hit us with cars and took the RBC's and WBC's from the remains? That first night in my new room I studied that booklet to ward off a wave of homesickness that threatened to engulf me.

And a few days later in our first classes I was thankful for my evening with the RBC's and WBC's. We began to fill our notebooks with an endless string of letters that were shorthand for a technique or a procedure. The particularly obscure abbreviations were explained, but the simple, everyday ones like RBC or CBC were not. Perhaps after generations of students had spent their first quarter mystified by HBC's, they decided that a brief note in our orientation booklet would save considerable confusion. I was so pleased that I was able to follow what was happening, that I knew the abbreviations. The look of dismay on the faces of students who obviously hadn't the faintest idea what RBC meant was poignant.

That orientation booklet was symbolic. It was the first time we realized it was important to notice *everything*, even the little box at the bottom of the page. We had to learn to become as observant, as meticulous as first-rank detectives. In years to come, when we would finally be examining animals on our own, there would be no one to tell us where to look for symptoms, no one to help point out a tiny irregularity that could be the clue to diagnosis.

The booklet was also our introduction to a new language, one that had evolved in a world where there's no time to waste on complete words. By the time we were fluent in vet, we'd be different people. As the first weeks passed and I became immersed in my new world, I had little time and attention for the old. I lost track of popular TV shows and the romances of the stars and of politics. In my last year of vet school when a man, learning I was from Ohio, asked me if there really was a WKRP radio station in Cincinnati I told him I wasn't sure—I was from the north of Ohio. It wasn't until weeks later that I learned he was talking about a popular TV show based on a fictitious Ohio radio station. He must have thought I was amazingly obtuse. We freshmen lived in our own insulated microcosm. We told jokes no one else could understand and we shared one another's anguish when an animal patient died. Our humor was black and bawdy, but at the same time we all began to experience a delicate sense of the mystery of man's binding link with animals.

PERFECTLY PORCINE

Like most freshmen, I spent the first few days of school learning my way around campus. I was living in a graduate student dorm and my new roommate was a law student from Ohio. I can still see the look on her face when I came back to the room after one of my first anatomy classes. I was carrying a metal box like a lunch pail. I swung it up onto my desk and she ambled over to watch me open it, expecting to share perhaps half a bologna sandwich or some Twinkies. But when I lifted the lid, she saw a tangle of small bleached bones. Each freshman was given a set to take home and study and, to my roommate's chagrin, I spent hours fondling the tubercles and protuberances on my bones, memorizing the names of all the parts of the dog skeleton.

The freshmen vet students took all their classes in the same building. Sisson Hall is an architecturally undistinguished structure that was one of the vet school's first. We might have been pleased to be a part of OSU's history if Sisson Hall hadn't been so grim and uncomfortable. All our classes were held in the auditorium, which was poorly lit and uncarpeted. The crowded seats were hard wood and perhaps they improved the moral fiber of generations of OSU's vet students who were going to have to practice without antibiotics and high-tech instruments. But we'd been spoiled as undergraduates and we bemoaned our lot. We spent freshman year yearning for the day when, as sophomores, we'd take our places in the brand-new auditorium, which had air-conditioning, carpeting, lighting with dimmers, sophisticated slide machines and comfortable seats. In the meantime, day after day we trooped determinedly into that old drafty auditorium for our classes in embryology, chemistry, anatomy, physiology, neurology and pharmacology.

When I look back, what I remember most clearly of those early days is not the courses but the other students. Perhaps because I was a newcomer, I was intensely aware of my colleagues. Most had gone to Ohio State University and they all knew one another. They greeted each other in the first days of classes with friendly hellos and hugs and they all seemed up to date on each others' lives right up until the beginning of the previous summer.

There were three freshmen from Miami University, only one of whom I knew, and that particular student wasn't really a close friend. He was a top graduate of Miami U. He'd had a 4.0 grade average. He had had the honor of being appointed a lab assistant in two courses—embryology and histology— when he was an undergraduate. He was the kind of person who spends graduation day up on the podium accepting awards.

I held none of this against him. Nonetheless our circles hadn't overlapped. I was your average fun-loving student. I worked hard enough to get decent grades—I graduated from Miami with a 3.4 grade average—but in all my four years of college I'd never really developed anything that could be called proper study habits. I crammed the night before a test, and it worked. My eleventh-hour style was to become one of my biggest problems as a freshman vet student.

Fortunately vet school encourages easy intimacy. Instead of sitting in lectures all day, taking notes in solitude, vet students work on projects together in the labs. When a cow carcass starts to fall on one of your colleagues or you dissect a piglet to discover that it's a hermaphrodite, it creates an inevitable closeness.

Anatomy class was an important part of that first quarter, not only because it was the foundation of much of what we would later learn, but also because it brought me one of my best friends, Donna. She had been a student at Miami University and at the first anatomy class we recognized each other and decided to join up as lab partners. Donna was a serious student and a good, steadying influence on me. She was living in a rooming house and we decided that, beginning with the second quarter, we'd get an apartment together. There would be no more alarming encounters with bleached bones for the law student, and I would have the support of living with a friend and fellow student. Donna and I were in many ways opposites. Where she was serious and studious, I tended to be more fun-loving. We were a good balance. I would drag Donna to parties and she would drag me back to the books. Wherever we went together, there was lots of laughter.

Among the best opportunities for meeting people at vet school were the OTS parties. OTS was a veterinary fraternity—a collection of rowdy guys who made it their business to provide comic relief from the rigors of studying. Early on in the quarter they held their annual ox roast. It drew a pretty wild collection of people and one of the wildest was a young woman who was square-dancing up a storm, attacking the reels and rounds with wild abandon. That's how Lesley and I met and she became another of my best friends. Lesley was a robust girl with long hair, red cheeks and a sunny expression who was full of adventure and enthusiasm. Lesley brought out the free spirit in me. She would try anything. She knew how to catch eels and how to cook venison. And she *surely* did know how to party.

Lesley was from New Hampshire and was one of the few out-of-state students. Because New Hampshire didn't have a vet school, they had an exchange program with OSU that had brought her to the wilds of Ohio. At the end of her education she was scheduled to pay a certain amount of money to the state of New Hampshire for her schooling, but in our senior year New Hampshire passed a retroactive bill providing for the tuition for vet students. So Lesley found herself at the end of senior year with something like a $30,000 surplus in her budget. It's to her credit that rather than squander the money on herself, she took Donna and me and a few other good friends out for a memorable drinking party that almost wiped out her windfall. Despite her fun-loving nature, Lesley was terribly smart and a good student. She just didn't seem to have to study as hard as others did to get good grades. Over the four years of vet school, we would make many trips, become champion Ping-Pong players, try parachute jumping and get into countless scrapes together.

My fellow freshmen proved to be an interesting group. Forty percent of us were women—the largest contingent of female vet students yet. We had a collective grade point average as undergraduates of 3.2. With a few exceptions, we were an especially bright class. It soon became clear to me that I was up against stiff competition, and in fact competition became a constant undercurrent in the four years of training.

The first freshmen to stand out were the odd ones. Like "the Rodent." She carried intensity to the extreme. The Rodent did nothing but study, and she did it so obsessively she soon became legend. She would bring a tape recorder to class and record every lecture and then have her tapes transcribed. She didn't want to miss a single "Um..." or a "Well..." The Rodent got her name because she was a nocturnal creature. She studied all night, most nights and, because the sun never touched her skin, she was astonishingly pale. In fact, if you encountered her in the hall late at night it was like seeing a ghost. It was rumored she lived on amphetamines. She would study in the Autotutorial Lab, or A/T Lab, and after that closed for the night she would find an empty office. I suppose there's a natural victim in every class and the Rodent was ours. The guys were constantly playing tricks on her. One night I was studying at the A/T lab and I heard a terrific noise that sounded like gunfire. I ran in the direction of the shots only to discover that someone had thrown a handful of firecrackers under the door of the office the Rodent was using. On quieter nights they would simply wear rubber horror masks and, in the small hours, press their faces against the glass window of the Rodent's sanctuary.

Ultimately, despite her intelligence and obsessive studying, the Rodent's neurosis did her in. In senior year she lost her temper when a professor told her she wouldn't be getting an A for the course and she picked up a paperweight from his desk and threw it at him. *Sic transit* Rodent.

There were times that freshman year when I felt as odd as the oddest of my fellows. Not because of curious study habits but because of my comparatively "citified" origins. Now Mentor, Ohio, is light-years away from Bloomingdale's. It's a typical middle-American bedroom suburb forty-five minutes driving time northeast of Cleveland on Lake Erie. But most of the vet students in my class grew up on farms and had had the kind of experience with animals you just can't get from books. They lived and breathed large animals and had been raising pigs and cows and sheep when I was still trying to convince my parents to buy me a puppy. Even Lesley and Donna had had more hands-on experience with animals than

I had, and though they were often helpful to me with suggestions and explanations, they couldn't always be on hand to bail me out.

One day in genetics class the professor gave a lecture on breeding animals for certain characteristics. I was, as usual, madly taking notes. Suddenly, the student to my right tapped me on the arm. "Sally," he said in a lazy accent that seemed to echo all the way down the Olentangy River, "that word there is 'porcine.'" I looked at my notes. I'd been writing "porsign." I had had no idea of what it meant, had assumed that it was some abstruse genetics term. "P-O-R-C-I-N-E." My friend spelled the word for me like an infinitely patient first-grade teacher and, as most of the students turned in their seats to laugh, he finished up his explanation, the words coming loud and clear and deliberate: "It means pig, Sally. P-I-G."

In another class there was a spirited discussion of the "abomasum," which everyone seemed to be on very familiar terms with. I had to nudge the farm boy next to me and ask, in a discreet whisper, what an abomasum was. He turned with astonishment to get a better look at me as he explained that an abomasum is the fourth stomach of a cow—something he'd probably known since the age of six. I was often the butt of jokes about the "city girl," but it was all in good fun. In fact most all of the students in my class got along wonderfully. We liked and respected one another and, aside from the never-ending, almost impersonal competition, we felt like willing prisoners on the same ship, eager for the day when we'd reach port and look back on the journey with nostalgia.

COWS' CRADLE

One of the first courses we took was called "Animal Restraints." It sounded like a variation on the honor code for cows and horses, but in fact it was a crash course in methods of getting animals to do what you want them to do by means of handholds or ropes. Mostly what you wanted them to do was lie down and be quiet so that you could examine them or administer drugs or take blood samples. Dogs and cats usually do this willingly and sometimes with enthusiasm. But cows, pigs and sheep have to be convinced. Sheep, as you might guess by their reputation, are pretty compliant. You can grab one from behind and sit it up on its haunches with ease. It stays so calm it looks idiotic. Cows and horses are difficult to maneuver for obvious reasons. The theoretical core of our restraints course was enabling a 100-pound woman to deck a 1,400-pound cow. It was a wonderful course to have in the beginning of vet school because it was so active and partici-patory that even when the animals weren't cooperating—in fact especially when they were at their most obstinate—we were being bound together as a group.

The foundation of effective restraint work is knot tying, and that's what we spent the beginning of the course doing. If you are a sailor and you need an extra hand in a boating emergency, you could do a lot worse than have vets as crew. We can tie bowlines, clove hitches, double half hitches and figure eights with our eyes closed. By the middle of the re-straints course, I could have rigged the HMS *Bounty* and then wrestled it onto dry land.

Once we knew our knots, we learned to use them on the animals. For most of us the most difficult technique was get-ting a cow to lie down on the ground in a relaxed but inviting position so that a vet could reach significant parts of its anat-omy. In order to do this you have to weave an intricate network of ropes around the cow's standing body. When you're done it looks as if you have a cow in a cat's cradle. Once that's achieved, you stand behind the animal and, with the end of the rope in your hand, you give a yank and the pressure of the rope at certain key points on the cow's anatomy forces it to fall to the ground where it lies docile, pretending nothing has happened.

After weeks of tying and weaving, we were ready to prove

our mettle as restrainers. Our restraints exam was a dread event made even worse by the fact that it was public. For days before you could spot the restraint students because we carried our ropes with us everywhere, obsessively tying and untying between classes, during meals and through lectures and conversations. We looked like a group of very slow campers. Donna and I worked for endless hours on our knots and late one night briefly considered testing various restraints on one another but neither of us was trusting enough to be the first to be trussed and so we had to abandon the notion of bondage.

For the first part of the test we had to stand in a row, ropes in hand. There were five "stations" with an instructor at each one. In our turn we would approach the station and the instructor would ask us to tie a particular knot. I stood anxiously, twisting my rope until it was my turn and I was asked to tie a bowline. After a few seconds' hesitation I did it correctly and breathed a huge sigh of relief. I got through my other four knots handily, though some of my colleagues stood mortified with their ropes at the moment of crisis, no doubt forgetting in their embarrassment even how to tie their shoelaces.

Once the knot test was over it was time for the animal work. The first student had to cast a cow and the anxiety was palpable. We were all facing the same hurdle. He positioned his cow and began to construct his trip device. Facing the cow, he ran the rope over the cow's back and under its chest, then up to the back again. He had to loop the rope into a sort of blanket stitch along the cow's spine until he reached its tail. Then it went down between the cow's rear legs and into the student's hands. The operation resembled a quilting bee at the OK Corral. The humor of the situation was, however, entirely lost on us. The student, brow furrowed, finally completed his weaving job and faced the cow's tail. He took the rope, gave it the requisite tug and nothing happened. We all held our breaths. He got a better grip on his end of the line and gave it all he had. With a powerful snap, he jerked the line and the first crucial knot he had tied came undone and the carefully constructed network dissolved. The rope slid off the cow and into a pile beneath its tail. We stood in silence until the instructor began to grin. As the cow watched, looking even more complacent than your average bovine, we began to laugh. The ice was broken and we went on to trip up cows and pigs and sheep with admirable success.

THE SCANDAL

Once the tentativeness of the first few days of school was gone, the atmosphere became charged with a spirit of intense competition that was to endure for the entire four years. It affected us all. I hated the competition and so did most everyone else, but like nuclear preparedness it seemed to take on a life of its own and we soon grew accustomed to it. Competition was a habit we had developed in our undergraduate days because of the scarcity of places in vet schools. Everyone knew he had to have the best grades, the best experience and most impressive record if he were to be accepted by a vet school. But once there, there was no real reason for the competition to continue. Only a small number of us went on to do postgraduate work, and our grades really had little effect on our job prospects—interviews and recommendations were far more important. There was a joke aimed at defusing the tension: "If you call the top graduate of your vet school class valedictorian, what do you call the bottom graduate? Doctor." But everyone had been competing for so long it would take more than a joke or simple common sense to stop it. If anything, it was more intense than ever: competition had become a reflex.

From one standpoint my lack of confidence at the beginning was a blessing. Knowing how bright and hard-working my fellow students were, I didn't feel I could ever successfully vie for top grades. I would work as hard as I could but I was going to be satisfied to be an average student. Anything beyond that would be a bonus. This gave me a relatively healthy perspective and removed me from the savagery of the fray.

One student who was tragically infected by the spirit of competition was Allen. Remembering him is remembering one of the worst ordeals I had to endure in vet school, because when all was said and done, Allen lost everything, and I'd played a part in his demise.

Allen was a standout from the first day. At least to the women. He was suavely handsome with remarkable self-assurance. Tall with dark brown hair and blue eyes, he had the slender body of a swimmer as opposed to the other halfback types who fit the "handsome guy" bill. He took particular care with his clothes and always looked, as my mother would say, "bandbox fresh." This was in stark contrast to the rest of us, who wore the same duds day after day. Why bother, most of us thought, if you're going to spend twelve hours up to your elbows in viscera?

After a few weeks it was clear that Allen was not only handsome, he was also smart. He'd graduated near the top of his undergraduate class and was getting high marks in vet school right from the beginning. The only flaw in his facade was his aloofness. He just didn't make friends. It wasn't as if he were one of the grinds. He just seemed to give off vibrations that said "stay away." So eventually we gave up and left Allen alone. He went his own way until one day when something happened that changed the way everyone thought of him and eventually altered the course of his career.

One of the most important freshman courses was anatomy. We spent six hours of class time on it a day and it took up most of our other waking thoughts as well. It was divided into two segments—small- and large-animal anatomy. In the fall we began with small animal. Three students were assigned to a dog and all quarter they worked on that dog—or, rather, dog carcass—memorizing every artery, vein and muscle, including origins and insertions, bone and nerve.

After you've passed the first quarter of vet school, if you fail a course you must stay back one year and retake the course.

It wasn't uncommon to see a vet student with a red name tag among your class of blue ones, identifying him as having failed a course and fallen back a year. If, however, you failed a course during the first quarter, the school felt you hadn't been able to prove yourself as bona fide vet material and you were forced to reapply to vet school the following year as a new applicant. One of the students in our anatomy class in freshman year flunked, was kicked out of school, reapplied the following year and was not readmitted. Losing one of our own so early sent a collective shiver through us.

In the winter we graduated to large-animal anatomy. Eight of us were assigned either a horse or a cow. The large animal carcasses were kept in huge walk-in coolers. They were hung from the ceiling on hooks and the hooks ran along tracks that left the cooler and went into the lab. At the beginning of each day's lab, we'd slide our animal out into a clear space and then the eight of us, usually four to a side, would begin whittling away, exploring the interior of our beast.

Our anatomy instructor, Dr. Wetmore, was a popular member of the faculty. He was relatively young—around thirty— and a good teacher. But he, unfortunately, was the beginning of Allen's end.

Anatomy tests were particularly dreaded, and after our first test we knew why. They included a practical as well as a written section. The written part was pro forma. But the practical section was nerve-racking. An open carcass of an animal would be put before you with questions pinned to various parts of its anatomy. You had to answer the questions and identify the parts as indicated. While this might not sound so difficult it was exceedingly tricky because no two animals are exactly alike inside. Moreover, when we practiced dissecting animals, we invariably developed slightly different techniques. These test carcasses might reveal all of an artery; another might reveal only a part. The animal in the test was one dissected by a stranger and, because you couldn't move the pins that sometimes obscured part of the carcass, you had to spend a few agonizing minutes looking for familiar interior landmarks before you could even think about the question. You had not only to know all the facts but you also had to be able to recognize things in place and, because of the internal variance, you couldn't rely on your textbook work to help you. You had really to have paid attention during the long hours of the lab.

The night before the test Dr. Wetmore went to work in the cooler marking them up for the next day. Two nights before the test, our last occasion to examine the animals, we all stayed at the lab until two or three in the morning when it closed, trying to fix in our minds the tiniest detail of their interior geography. Donna and I spent hours and hours quizzing one another on anatomy until visions of arteries danced in our heads.

On the night before our first anatomy test, after the animals were prepared, Dr. Wetmore closed the cooler door around midnight and, for reasons of his own, put a small piece of tape on to seal it, right near the floor. The next morning, before the test, he noticed that the tape was broken.

As far as we were concerned, the morning was uneventful. Dr. Wetmore said nothing about the broken tape and simply took note of the test results.

When it came time for the second test, Dr. Wetmore tried a new approach. We spent our feverish evening studying and the next night he marked the animals as usual, but instead of using the tape on the door, he decided to sleep in the lab himself to keep an eye on things. He obviously suspected someone was breaking into the cooler before the test and this time he planned to surprise him. He took a blanket into the corner and settled in for the night. How peculiar he must have felt lying alone in that cold, tiled room, surrounded by stainless-steel dissection tables, waiting for a furtive visitor. At about three in the morning he was awakened by the creak of the lab door and the soft glow of a flashlight. He must have been holding his breath, waiting for the light of the cooler to illuminate the culprit. Who would be so bold? But when the door opened Dr. Wetmore must have been as much confused as surprised. He waited until the person began to write down the numbers and their placement on the carcasses, then swung open the cooler door and confronted not a student but Dr. B., a young woman who was a professor of biochemistry. Amazed, Dr. Wetmore asked her what she was doing. Dr. B. would say only that she was helping a student study.

When the results of the second test came in, most everyone had missed one question—the same question. When the carcass was pulled out of the cooler in the morning, one of the markers had been moved. Obviously surprised, Dr. B. had disturbed a marker on the carcass by accident, perhaps when she was caught by Dr. Wetmore. So everyone was tripped up. Everyone, that is, except one student: Allen, who knew where the marker was *supposed* to be. It was suddenly clear to Dr. Wetmore who Dr. B. was helping. Allen was working in Dr. B.'s course as an assistant, perhaps doing more than simply assisting her with her slides.

OSU has an honor code. It is taken very seriously. At our freshman orientation we were given booklets describing the code and were quizzed on the material. One of its tenets is that if someone is caught cheating, he or she must be reported within twenty-four hours. For some reason—perhaps Dr. Wetmore's reluctance to implicate a colleague—Allen wasn't reported and no one but Dr. Wetmore was the wiser about Allen's peculiar study habits.

By sophomore year there were occasional rumors about Allen. I had heard he'd been found cheating, but I didn't pay too much attention. Idle gossip, I thought. But when it came time for our cardiology final, the professor announced that we were to sit in assigned seats, which was unusual as we had never been given specific places for any test before. We all looked at one another questioningly as we took our places. Allen, whose last name was near the very beginning of the alphabet, would wind up right in the front row. He was the only one to protest the arrangement and the professor had to insist that he come down from the back and take his place. This incident kept the rumor mill in business for weeks afterward. What people couldn't understand was why someone as smart as Allen would cheat when he really had no need to. I didn't know what to believe, but I was so preoccupied by my own work that I gave it little thought.

It was in my junior year that I became directly involved in Allen's life.

I was taking a digestive exam and it was an essay test. Because I wrote fairly lengthy answers and because I always used to read and reread them to be sure they were right, I was often the last one to finish. So it was with digestive. I was sitting in the front row and when I lifted my head and gathered my papers there seemed to be no one else in the room. But when I headed to the back to add my test to those on the table I saw someone standing at the table writing furiously. He was looking at other papers and making additions to his own. It was Allen. When he realized someone else was in the room he stopped abruptly. Giving me a big friendly smile, he said he'd forgotten to write his name on his paper.

I didn't want to believe that Allen was a cheat, but there was no eluding the fact that his actions were highly suspect. As everyone had handed in their work, and for fear that Allen might return and continue to "write his name" on the pages, I took it upon myself to collect the papers and take them all into the professor. "Thanks, Sally," he said, "but you didn't have to make a hand delivery." I could see he was wondering what was going on so I told him I thought it would be a good idea for him to be on hand occasionally while we were being tested. I didn't want to be more explicit than that. "Allen?" he asked, giving me a searching look. Suddenly I had the feeling I was getting involved in something I'd just as soon leave alone. But the professor had had his eye on Allen and this was the opportunity he'd been looking for.

"Sally," he told me, gesturing for me to sit down. "Let me

talk to you for a minute." My heart sank. "You have a responsibility to yourself and your other classmates to report
Allen if you saw him cheating. I know there've been rumors
about him, but no one has actually caught him in the act.
Now it seems you have. You can't afford to let this slide and
I don't want you to." Then he added, "Did you know there
are vets out there who cheated as students and now they're
cheating as vets—doing one little thing after another to make
an extra dollar or to avoid the hard work they should be putting
in? Allen could turn out to be the kind of vet who puts a coin
under an animal's stomach when he X-rays it and then tells
its owner he has to operate to remove a foreign body. I don't
want to teach students like that and I don't want to graduate
vets like that."

The last thing I wanted to do was report Allen, but it
seemed I had no choice. After all, if he was cheating, it was
unfair to all of us, since we were often graded on a curve. I
had never thought about the kind of vet Allen might be. We
were all so engrossed in being students that we didn't often
consider the life ahead of us as vets in the real world. I felt
very alone. But, on reflection and after long supportive talks
with Donna, I realized I should have the courage to at least
report what I'd seen. I wouldn't be making the final decision
on Allen. His fate would be up to the student council.

The procedure was gruesome. First I had to write a brief
description of what I had witnessed. That was difficult enough,
but the worst part was having to appear before the council,
in front of the Dean, with Allen sitting in, and describe again
how I'd seen him writing on his paper and comparing it to
the others. I was so upset I was near tears. I had to make
myself think of him as someone who would cheat vulnerable
people who loved their pets, who would fail to act in the best
interests of the animals he treated. Even then, it was an ordeal.

I made my presentation and then Allen got up to defend
himself. He claimed he was only writing his name on the top
of his paper and going over his grammar. When asked, I said

I was fairly sure he had written more than a single word or two—that he indeed looked to be writing whole paragraphs. Everyone in the room seemed convinced that Allen was cheating—after all, there had already been lots of suspicion about him. Yet because there was no hard evidence beyond my testimony, he got away with it once again. When I could finally get some distance from the experience, I was glad I had reported him. I felt it was something that should be done if the honor code could continue to be effective.

Finally, in senior year, Allen met his Waterloo. We were taking what were called "latent-image" exams. The sheet on which you marked your answers was treated with a chemical so that, when you used a particular pen with yellow ink to indicate your choice, additional information appeared on the page. The questions built on one another and had many parts. For example, one scenario might open with a dog's being brought in because it had diarrhea. You had to choose a course of action. If you chose to examine the stool, the answer sheet indicated this was a correct response and that the dog had hookworms, and what would you do next? If, faced with the presenting diarrhea, you chose instead to give the dog an angiogram, the paper would tell you that, "Oops! The dog died and you're faced with a malpractice suit." Despite the tension, there would always be nervous giggles, usually from the very people who were killing their animals.

When the answer sheets were being graded, the grader noticed that on one particular test many of the answers had a peculiar feature. Instead of just one bold mark at a "Yes" or a "No," there were often tiny marks on both possible answers. It was obvious that the test taker had tried to mark just enough of the answer to see if he could read whether or not he had the right one. If the beginning of a "Y" appeared, he knew this was a "Yes" answer, but if the beginning of an "N" appeared, that answer was abandoned and the student chose the other option.

The astute grader took the test to the professor and it turned out to be Allen's. Enraged at yet another violation of the honor code by this student who'd been flouting the system for four years, the professor went to the honor committee. This time there was positive evidence of the intent to cheat and Allen was expelled. So after nearly four full years of work Allen achieved nothing. The terrible irony was that he had never *needed* to cheat. If it hadn't been for his obsession with always getting the best mark, the highest grade, he would be out practicing right now. And, after all, even though we so often forgot it, that was the whole point.

DUCK SHOTS

There is no one more trusting than a freshman. Tell her she must wear pink shoelaces and carry senior books and she will. At most schools freshman hazing is the domain of fraternities and sororities. At vet school it assumed a medical cast. When they told us to report to the infirmary for our rabies shots, and fools that we were, we were there in line with our arms held docilely out.

Much to most people's surprise, despite a recent outbreak of the disease carried largely by raccoons, rabies in pets has not been a major problem in this country. Still it's probably the most feared disease because its symptoms are so dreadful and phrases like "vicious as a rabid dog" have made it seem common and terrifying. Most kids spend a small percentage of their childhood discussing whether they'd rather have the required nine rabies shots in their stomachs or freeze to death. Some people have only to see a bit of foam on a dog's mouth to panic. Certainly rabies is a serious disease because it can be fatal to all warm-blooded animals, including humans. If rabies is suspected, a ten-day observation period must be observed. If the pet shows progressive neurological signs, it must be euthanized and its brain sent to a lab for analysis. But most cases of rabies are contracted not from household pets but from wild animals, particularly, in this country, skunks, raccoons, bats and foxes. The law in most places, except, curiously enough, New York City, demands that pets be inoculated against rabies so that if a pet is bitten by a rabid raccoon there will be less chance that the animal becomes infected.

Vets, in the course of their work, can be easily exposed to rabies and so one of the early events in freshman life is to get a rabies vaccination. We were excited. This was confirmation that soon we would be working with flesh-and-blood animals.

The principle of the rabies vaccine is that it encourages a body to build up an immunity to a specific disease. A tiny portion of the virus is injected into a healthy body. The presence of the virus stimulates the production of antibodies that will remain in the body for a long time. It's those antibodies that will offer protection if the person is ever bitten. Even if you've had the vaccine, however, you're not completely protected. You still have to get a certain number of those dreaded shots, but not the full complement, and your reaction is supposedly limited. The vaccine we took was grown in duck embryos.

The duck embryo vaccine was considered relatively safe, or safe enough for freshmen, I guess. Certainly we didn't know enough to be nervous about it. One after another we rolled up our sleeves. But word was beginning to spread that we had to wait for twenty minutes after the shot to see if we developed any reaction. An anaphylactic reaction is life-threatening and, should one develop, we'd need an immediate shot of epinephrine—the treatment. There were lots of jokes about shooting on sight any freshman who started to foam at the mouth and bite other students. Fortunately, no one in the class had a reaction and we all trooped cheerfully off to classes.

The next morning I woke up to find an arm the size of Arnold Schwarzenegger's beside me. Much to my astonishment, it was attached to my body. Too much note-taking, I thought, until I noticed the strange red bumps that covered it. Despite its impressive size, the arm was not very useful, and I was glad that it was my left. I dragged it over to the phone and called the infirmary. "What reactions can you get from the duck embryo shot?" I asked. "Mainly anaphylaxis." "What does that do to you?" "Kills you." So this is how it ends, I thought. All that studying and hoping and hard work, only to be felled by a rabid duck embryo. Well, at least I wouldn't have to stick around and figure out how to get this giant arm into a sleeve. Or would I? "How fast?" I asked the infirmary. At last they realized I wasn't an idle caller and told me to come over immediately. "I'll be bringing an arm," I told them and hung up.

I savored that walk across campus as if it were my last, which I thought it might well be. They at least could have warned us we were risking our lives by entering this profession, I thought. I wonder how many they lose each year to this procedure? Who would get my old room? I was sorry I hadn't cleaned it before I left. My mother would be horrified when she came to pick up my things.

"Hives," the doctor said as he examined the humongous arm. "You'll live." This was good news except that it turned out the arm would live, too, and we'd be living together. He gave me some antihistamine to cut down on the itching but it did little good. Every time something touched that arm it itched like crazy. For the next five days I alternated between itching and sleeping off the effects of the antihistamine in class. Surely I had enough obstacles to success in vet school without my own arm turning against me.

When it came time to get another rabies shot, I was no longer a freshman and I'd lost my trusting nature. "No," I said. But it turned out that they'd developed a new vaccine called "human diploid" that they were positive would cause no reaction. After considerable convincing, I held out my arm and took it like a woman. The next morning I woke to a normal-sized arm and, in a few weeks, an immunity to rabies.

THE ENDOCRINE CRISIS

I learned two things in vet school.

First, I absorbed an enormous volume of material. Lectures, notes, slides, text, procedures and the dynamism of living things from protozoa to pigs became part of my store of knowledge. These bits of information produced unconscious reflexes. If I heard someone hum "Baa-baa, Black Sheep," I wondered what breed they were singing about. Instead of saying "I have to use the ladies' room," I began to slip into the clinical: "Excuse me. My bladder is full." I could look at certain pieces of modern art and discover an excellent example of the pattern of Ostertagia, a bovine parasite, or perhaps the manifestation of sarcoptic mange in dogs. All this information was turning me into a medical person—more specifically, into a vet.

The other education I was getting involved the very process of learning. I was forced to develop a whole new way to study. My eleventh-hour cram style had to go by the boards. The volume of material was simply too great. Not only that, there were so many tests I'd often have two the same day and some weeks included as many as seven quizzes or tests. It was overwhelming. When you add to the pressure of the work itself the fact that the other students were so dedicated and so smart, and so willing to study night and day, it becomes clear that I was in deep waters. I felt like the only one who hadn't been the valedictorian of my undergraduate class and who had never worked with large animals. It was a rude awakening.

And there was a special distraction that started at the end of that first quarter. I met Dave, who was to become my boyfriend and best friend through most of vet school. I was at a party in an apartment complex and had no sooner walked in the door than a tall, blond guy said, "Hi, Sally." I knew I'd never met him—I would have remembered a guy *that* cute!—so I was a bit off guard. It turned out he had asked one of my classmates about me. We had chatted for a few minutes when someone announced that more ice was needed in order to continue the revelry. Dave's apartment was in the same complex so he was enlisted to provide ice. But as he was already serving as bartender, he gave me the keys to his apartment to fetch the supplies. By the time I left on my mission, I'd already had a bit more than my share of Southern Comfort and I found it a real challenge to pick out Dave's door. As I walked from apartment to apartment, trying the key, doors opened in my wake and heads peered after me. One of those bewildered faces called to me and wound up directing me to Dave's apartment. But in the course of giving directions he told me he was from my hometown so we spent a cheerful time catching up on old Mentor, Ohio.

Back at the party, Dave was growing concerned. I don't know if I was becoming more attractive the longer I stayed away or if he was simply worried about giving his keys to a tipsy woman he hardly knew. Anyhow, by the time a search party had been organized and Dave had found me, he'd decided he'd like to date me and that's how it began.

Fortunately, Dave was a year ahead of me and that turned out to be a lucky break: whenever I was having trouble understanding something I could turn to him. Our dating life centered around studying. We'd meet at the A/T Lab, at the library, at his apartment or mine to work together. Some of the time we got work done. But sometimes high spirits would possess us and we'd end up laughing and joking and moving on to a diversion like a beer or a snack at one of the millions of nearby fast-food emporiums. The only drawback to my relationship with Dave was that it inevitably put a subtle strain on my friendship with Donna. Donna and I had always studied together. Now, more and more, I was spending that time with Dave. Try as I might, I was no longer a constant in her life. The *only* constant in all our lives at vet school seemed to be studying.

The turning point in the revolution of my relatively relaxed study habits came during the spring quarter of my freshman year in my endocrine course.

Ohio State followed the "systems" approach to veterinary education. Most schools teach animal by animal so that they'd offer a course on equine or bovine diseases or diseases of the cat or of the dog. We had a certain number of those courses as electives but instead of studying a particular animal we studied the systems of all animals—system by individual system. We had courses in digestive, musculoskeletal, integument, respiratory, endocrine, cardiovascular and urinary systems, among others. We would begin with an example of the normal anatomy and physiology of, say, the digestive tract, and then go on to what can go wrong, including congenital abnormalities, infectious diseases, metabolic diseases, trauma, cancer and so on, and finally we'd learn how to treat them. The virtue of the systems approach is that it's so comprehensive and completely rational—you discover how all the parts are connected as an integrated system—but it can be confusing.

One of the major courses in freshman year was endocrine. It was a study of the endocrine system, which consists of glands that send substances into the bloodstream which then regulate various body functions. When the endocrine system malfunctions, diseases such as Cushing's disease and diabetes can occur. We learned all about hyperthyroid cats and hypothyroid dogs. Cats who are hyperthyroid—and it's a condition that mainly afflicts older cats—typically drink a lot, urinate a lot, have diarrhea and are usually ravenously hungry, with thin faces and prominent jawbones, and they are wildly hyperactive. Dogs, usually struck with the opposite of hyperthyroid, hypothyroid, are fat and lethargic. Their coats thin and they develop ratlike hairless tails. Because hypothyroid dogs like to cozy up to any heat source, they are known as "heat seekers."

The professor who taught endocrine had a perfectly functioning thyroid himself. In fact, it was his single flaw as a teacher. His thyroid kept his metabolism on such an even keel that his delivery was in strict monotone and we had to fight to stay awake in his class.

We had three tests in the course. For the first I thought I

was well prepared. I'd studied with Donna and we'd gone over all the material thoroughly. But when I sat down to take the test, my confidence vanished. This was a whole new approach. Instead of having one right answer, all the questions had a problem you had to solve before you could go on to give the answers, and parts of the test were interrelated: if you got part A wrong, you couldn't possibly succeed with parts B and C. I struggled through, telling myself I was doing fine, that I was well prepared—I had, after all, studied for an evening and a half—and I was sure to do well enough.

When the grades came back a third of the class had failed, including me. I can still remember the tight, sinking feeling in the pit of my stomach when I saw my grade. I'd never failed a test before and I was devastated. That so many others had failed was no comfort. After all, Donna had passed. It was difficult to recapture my natural optimism, and as I walked across campus the day endocrine grades were posted, I chatted and laughed with my friends, but the seed of potential failure had been planted somewhere in me and I couldn't ignore it. Even Dave, with his assurances that endocrine was a killer course, couldn't console me.

As the second test approached, I realized I was going to have to work harder than ever. I needed a new plan of attack. I disciplined myself to set aside regular study hours when I worked on nothing but endocrine. And, to my surprise, I found that once I got into the material, I enjoyed the work and the feeling of mastery. I tried to make associations with everything I was learning so all the endless facts and details would stick with me. For example, Cushing's disease in dogs: Cushing's is a malfunction of the adrenal gland in which it releases too much cortisone. Its symptoms include excessive urination and water consumption, thinning hair, a pendulous belly, an enlarged liver, thin skin and comedones. Comedones, or blackheads, are what stuck in my mind. There's no doubt that dogs are capable of embarrassment. Some are mortified by a haircut, some are wretched when they have to wear a protective Elizabethan collar to keep them from worrying an injured part of their body. But blackheads! Were they self-conscious? Did they decide to limit their garbage-can pickings to lean meat and poultry and skip all chocolate and soft drinks? It was an unforgettable symptom. Surely on the next test I would do well.

But when the second test was given, I failed that too. This was a crisis of major proportions. My confidence was shattered. Could it be that my initial fears about vet school were proving true? Was it possible I just couldn't do the work? I knew people could flunk out of vet school. I'd already seen it happen in my own class. Would I be the next to go? I was in a panic.

The third and last test was to be given right after Memorial Day. I had planned to go home and visit my parents over that weekend but now that was out of the question. I had to stay on campus and study. The term at Ohio State for serious cramming was "gunning." Like gunning a car at the start of the race, it was a kind of mental acceleration. Over that Memorial Day weekend, and in fact for weeks previous, I gunned for that test. Ordinarily, this would have been a dramatic effort for me. But it was made even more difficult because suddenly we were having tests regularly in most of our courses. I was like a novice juggler who'd just mastered two balls and now was being tossed a half dozen.

The pressure was on. It began to seem that I'd just finished taking one quiz—I'd literally just leave the classroom—when I'd have to find a quiet place so I could start working for the next one. I couldn't just let everything else go to gun for my upcoming endocrine test. For the first time, studying was all-preoccupying. Even Dave was beginning to feel left out. He had friends who were dating women in my class and they all seemed to find the time to get together. I kept telling him to wait until next quarter. It became a bittersweet joke between us.

Finally it was time to take that last endocrinology test. By then I was so used to relentless studying that it didn't seem like I was giving the extra effort that I'd given for the previous test. I was like a war horse who just kept charging at the sound of the trumpet without reflection or deliberation.

I did have a treat planned for right afterward: Dave and I and Dave's roommate, Brownie, were going parachuting. Dave had done it before and I had always wanted to try. I had mentioned it once to my parents and they were horrified, but I was determined. Now I would have my chance. We thought of rounding up some additional recruits, so right before that last endocrine test I stood up in class and announced our plans and said that anyone who wanted to join us was welcome. The professor suggested that I might well save myself a good deal of anxiety by parachuting *before* the test. We all laughed— no one louder than myself—but I couldn't help wondering if he was convinced I'd be better off in the hospital! Nonetheless, exhilarated at the thought of drifting effortlessly through the blue Ohio skies, I ripped through the questions and dashed off to my fantastic adventure. But as I dropped into the sky, my heart in my mouth, trying to remember the proper position for landing in electric wires and the proper position for landing in trees and how fast to count before I pulled open my chute, I did think for an instant that my endocrine worries might shortly be over.

It seemed to take forever but finally the grades came in. I was so nervous I couldn't believe my eyes. I'd gotten an "A"! My sense of relief and accomplishment was enormous. The professor passed me in the course with a generous "C," even after two failures on three tests. I suppose he knew I had worked like a demon, even for that second, failed test, and he was partly grading me for effort. To this day, I'm thankful to him.

In retrospect, failing those two tests was the best, if most frightening, thing to happen to me in vet school. It gave me a new seriousness about studying. I had come too close to the jaws of student death. Eleventh hour was no longer soon enough for me.

When word of my "A" in endocrine circulated, Dave, his roommate, Donna, Lesley and a whole enthusiastic group of us went into town to celebrate. We threw even our limited caution to the winds and ordered the flaming drinks that were the pub's specialty. Forgetting about his mustache, Dave tucked into a flaming drink, and seconds later, amid howls of laughter, I was dabbing his face with a wet napkin, extinguishing the blaze. In the giddy madness of that moment I finally felt the terrible anxiety of my endocrine crisis—and of that whole arduous freshman year—begin to dissolve. I'd gotten through, I'd done all right.

AMBULATORY SUMMER

PIG NUMBER 83

Freshman year was over at last. After a tentative beginning, the whole class had fallen into place. No longer those nervous creatures worrying over RBC's and HBC's, we were now nearly sophomores. We knew who was class brain and who was class clown. We could find our way around campus without a map and equally effortlessly around the interior of a cow. But we still had a lot to learn. About pigs, for example.

Most people have used the expression "squealed like a stuck pig" but few understand exactly how a stuck pig squeals. My innocence about pig squealing was lost during the summer between my freshman and sophomore year of vet school.

When exams were over and grades in, the students scattered. Some worked in the veterinary hospital at OSU as work-study students while others worked in vet practices to gain hands-on experience. A number of my classmates worked in non-vet-related jobs just to raise tuition money. A few free spirits simply packed their bags and boxes of bones and traveled across the country looking for nonacademic adventure. I had originally thought I'd go back home to Mentor and get a job, but instead I decided to stay in my apartment in Columbus, get a job in town and tag along on the school's "ambulatory" service in order to increase my farm-animal experience.

Ohio State has two ambulatory services: one is at the vet clinic in Columbus and the other is based at a clinic in Marysville, a town some thirty miles from Columbus. Most students work on the ambulatory service for the summer prior to their senior year and for a rotation during senior year itself. It's the first big chance to experience what our professors have constantly been threatening us with: field conditions. The students ride with one of three Ohio State vets who travel the circuit from farm to farm.

I decided to unofficially join the ambulatory service two years early because of my large-animal inexperience. I was tired of being nearly the only one in the class who hadn't stripped a mammary gland or palpated a bovine ovary. Since I had three years of vet school ahead of me, and two of them before I would experience ambulatory, I decided it would make a lot of sense to try and get a jump on things. I was going to make up for being the class "city kid" in one summer of deep barnyard immersion.

Ambulatory service does its regular rounds during the day, so if I wanted to tag along with the vets I'd have to find a paying job at night. I'd never waitressed before but it seemed like a good option so I went to a popular restaurant in Columbus, the Brown Derby, and asked for a job. They had all their summer help already but they did have an opening for a cocktail waitress in their bar, the Luv Pub. This sounded ominous to me. If the restaurant jobs had been filled so fast, why hadn't the Luv Pub locked in their staff? Why, for that matter, had someone named it "The Luv Pub"? But I took a deep breath and said I'd take the job.

Life at the Lub Pub, to my surprise and delight, was great fun. I'd arrive at about four or five in the afternoon and work until three the next morning. I got a quick education in mixology and learned the quarterbacking moves that are necessary to transport trays of drinks through large crowds intent on fun. Cocktail waitressing didn't seem like work to me because there was always a nice crowd of people and a good band.

Best of all, I got to know people who existed in a different world, friends who had nothing to do with veterinary medicine, and it did me good. It reintroduced me to civilization, or at least the peculiar civilization of the dancing late-night brew and burger crowd.

Shuttling between the carefree world of the Luv Pub and the muck and medicine world of ambulatory made for an unforgettable summer. There was the contrast in uniforms, for example. As a cocktail waitress I dressed in modest black nylon with a frilly white apron. At the end of a shift, when I'd arrive home tired and happy, my uniform would reek of cigarette smoke and old beer. Despite these drawbacks, the Luv Pub duds had it all over the ambulatory togs.

My first day on ambulatory was a short course in field fashions for vets. Before we climbed into the pickup trucks we climbed into our coveralls. On top of the coveralls went our big high rubber boots. We wore stethoscopes around our necks and our horse leads dangled from one of our pockets. In our other pockets we carried our little black books, which provided drug dosages and other crucial information and which we used for taking notes. Fully rigged, we'd gained about ten pounds in body weight and about ten degrees in body temperature. By the end of rounds, reeking of manure and sweat and whatever else we'd encountered in the various barnyards, the stale odor of the Luv Pub nylon seemed like Chanel No. 5.

The first few days of ambulatory went off without a hitch. A farmer would call us about a case of milk fever in a cow or we'd come to scrape a horse's hoof to check for an abscess. They were simple, routine cases but I loved every call we made because I was getting a chance at hands-on experience with large animals, which is something that, fortunately, I managed to elude at the Luv Pub. I was becoming confident around cows, skilled with sheep and quite at home with horses. And then, very early in the summer, the day came for pig sticking.

The farmers who sought our services were used to students.

I suppose they thought of us as a necessary evil. I also think they savored our ignorance. But most often they barely noticed us. Until we threw them a curve ball by being women. I couldn't help but contrast my two summer occupations and the way my "customers" saw me in each: the same farmer who would have laughed and joked with me about being a vet student if he'd stopped in for a cold one at the Luv Pub took a pretty jaundiced view of me working on his animals. After all, that was his *livelihood*.

Pig sticking involves assembling a herd of pigs, grabbing them one by one and taking a blood sample from each. The pigs are relentlessly uncooperative and seem to be under the misapprehension that people in rubber clothes holding syringes are torturing them for pleasure. The main point of pig sticking is to test each porker's blood for common diseases. The other minor point seems to be to test the ears and patience and stamina of anyone who claims they want to work with animals. The fact that pig sticking must be done on a regular basis would weaken the resolve of any wavering vet students.

The farmers seemed sadistically happy to see us arrive for pig sticking. Testing pigs is low on the lineup of desirable ways to spend the afternoon. Pigs are intensely physical, nervous, noisy and ungrateful. Despite the fact that a pig may already have been stuck a half dozen times in his life, he never accepts his fate gracefully. A pig gives blood under protest.

When we arrived at the farm on that first day, the farmer looked me over. I could practically hear the wheels spinning in his head as I watched his expression change from mild skepticism to gleeful if subdued anticipation. Like a Christian alone in the Roman arena waiting for the lions to be released, I saw my audience gear up for fun. Amusing enough to watch big strapping male students grab the pigs but watching a girl do it would be better than a double feature.

The pigs were waiting for us in a small corral. There were about two hundred of them and you could tell by the way they muscled their way around the paddock that they would brook no nonsense. As the farmer settled into a comfortable position leaning against the fence and smiling to himself with ill-concealed pleasure at this opportunity to watch mud wrestling in his own front yard, we waded into the sea of cruising pink submarines.

The experienced vet showed us how to grab and hold a pig while another student takes a blood sample. Child's play. You just try to grab a few hundred pounds of screaming bacon and use every ounce of strength you can muster to convince the animal to stay in one place for a few seconds so someone can shove a ten-inch needle into his neck and draw blood. Of course there are some instruments that have been developed to help you achieve your goal. Once you've selected your pig you use a pole with a wire loop attached to help reel him in. This is called a snare and looks like a butterfly net without the net. You swing it over the pig's snout and then, trying to keep your mind free of rancor, you pull the wire that tightens around the snout until the pig gets the idea. It was at this point in the procedure—the timeless moment where snare and venous stick converged in an explosion of movement and sound—that I learned how a stuck pig squeals. Imagine that you are in a tunnel that stretches from Jacksonville, Florida, to Tacoma, Washington, and that tunnel is filled with eighteen-wheelers doing eighty. Suddenly in the same split second every single semi slams on its brakes. That's what it sounds like when you stick a pig.

After a few tries, it was obvious I wasn't champion pig-grabbing material. Every pig I grabbed immediately remembered a previous engagement. The pigs that accepted my snare did so only fleetingly. This is what happens, I thought, when a wallflower goes berserk. But it was soon clear that I wasn't a total washout: I would make my name as a sticker. In order to bleed a pig you take the ten-inch needle and, while someone else clutches the porker, you make what is called a "blind stick" into the neck at a certain angle. It's called "blind" because pigs have such fat necks you can't be absolutely positive you're sticking the right place until you actually see the blood in your syringe. We were aiming for the anterior vena cava. I'd plunge in the needle and then slowly begin to withdraw it, keeping suction on the syringe. If I'd hit the right place, my syringe would begin to fill with blood. I seemed to have a knack for pig bleeding and I hit the right spot almost invariably. While being an accomplished pig-sticker may not be a ticket to media superstardom, I nonetheless found that a lot of pleasure accompanied the discovery of my gift. Even the farmer, surveying the circus from fence-side, seemed impressed.

By the time we finished bleeding all those pigs, it was hard to tell the porkers from their guests. We were covered with mud and whatever else falls on the ground when a pig is finished with it. We'd been working in the hot sun for hours in our coveralls and boots and we were sweating like pigs, to use another expression that assumed a special meaning for me that day. We were used to the smell but the noise was something else. It was so intense and unrelenting that our spirits were bludgeoned. But we had our precious vials of blood and we piled back into the pickup truck, bade the vastly amused farmer and his herd farewell and headed back to the clinic.

I was feeling pretty smug on the ride back to the lab. I was accomplishing just what I'd wanted to that summer. I'd become a master at stripping milk glands. I could distinguish pig breeds by their ears and their colors: a Poland China is black with white spots at the feet and tail, a Chester White is all white and so is a Yorkshire but a Yorkshire has erect rather than floppy ears. I was beginning to feel knowledgeable around large animals, and *now* it turned out that I had the gift of pig-sticking.

After a long, dusty ride, we arrived at the lab and the technician began to spin down the blood. I'd never seen this procedure before and I made an eager audience. The blood is in a glass vial and the vial is put in a centrifuge that spins it until it separates into two parts: a clot and serum. The serum contains the antibodies, and once the blood is spun down, it is sent off to a lab for analysis. Spinning down the blood is one of those jobs that looks interesting the first time you watch it but achieves new heights of tedium when you're faced with a few hundred vials of pig blood that must pass through your hands. Because it was new to me, I was eager to give it a try so I asked the technician if I could spin down a vial.

I put the vial in the centrifuge and spun it down. It was amazing to watch it separate into a yellow and a red band. When it was fully separated, I took the clot with a sort of giant tweezer from the vial and bent over to throw it into the waste can. But as I bent I accidentally tipped the vial and the serum from pig Number 83 was soon spreading into what looked like a swamp of chicken bouillon on the floor at my feet. I looked at the empty vial in my hand and at the faces of the vet and the technician, who stood frozen, mesmerized by my accident, appreciating its implications. At last the silence was broken. "You're a fine pig-sticker, Sally," the vet said, "but you're going to have to work on your lab technique."

Back into our coveralls, back into the pickup, back the twenty miles to the farm, back to pig Number 83. Through my apologies and embarrassment the good-natured vet reminded me of something that I'd certainly experienced but had never articulated. Everything you do in vet school, every technique, is new. Whether it's spinning down blood or palpating an ovary or restraining a cow, it's a *new* skill. You get used to watching people doing these things effortlessly but you have to remember they've been doing them for years. When you start out, you're clumsy and awkward and nothing comes naturally. You must be patient with yourself. His encouragement boosted my flagging spirits and I girded my loins for the resticking of Pig Number 83.

Early the next morning, after a hasty transformation from Miss Piggy to the pride of the Luv Pub, I had just enough energy to bake some cookies for the vet and the technician. I gave them each a box with a card that said, "From Pig Number 83."

SOPHOMORE YEAR

FLYING HORSES

When we began our sophomore year we were, in our collective approach to veterinary medicine, sophomoric. Which is to say we were opinionated and self-assured but totally lacking experience or maturity. By the end of that second year most of us would retain our brave fronts but, humbled by time in the trenches, we'd be less arrogant and more aware that veterinary medicine is an art as well as a science.

Our freshman year had been devoted to basic courses in anatomy, physiology, chemistry, pharmacology, pathology, embryology and the like. These crucial subjects were building blocks but they were about as interesting as a building block can be, which isn't very. Sophomore year we began to get perspective—some sense of direction and of what the future would hold for us. It wasn't until sophomore year that we began to get some firsthand experience with animals in treatment. We had some of our own instruments and we finally began to think of ourselves as vets. This was largely due to the connection we began to develop with the clinics.

From the point of view of the patients and their owners, the OSU vet clinics functioned just like a neighborhood veterinary hospital. When your pet was sick or needed a shot or had had an accident, you'd go to the clinic. There was a waiting room filled with people and their pets. If the animals had problems requiring a hospital stay, they'd be admitted to the

65

wards. The difference between the clinic and the average vet's office was size and intensity. At OSU the waiting room was about as large as you'd find in an emergency hospital—three or four times the average vet's waiting room.

The intensity came from the students themselves. We were everywhere. We about doubled the human population at the clinic at any given time. We were always hovering in the background. We'd accompany a vet when a pet was examined, we'd observe procedures, we'd do routine work on the animals. Our sophomore courses—respiratory, cardiology, urinary— were beginning to prove practical. Often a professor would mention a particular disease such as a PDA—patent ductus arteriosis—that you could encounter in, say, Ward 6. We would troop over to the wards after classes, read the appropriate charts, pull out our stethoscopes and listen to the classic "machinery-type murmur" which is associated with this congenital abnormality.

This was a long way from amoebas and chemicals.

At the same time, we were grass green. We knew a lot but our bodies were forever betraying us. We had no grace, no rhythm. For example, there was the day we had to give our first shot. Now for many of the people in our class it wasn't a first shot by a long shot. Some students had had experience in vets' offices and on their own families' farms where they'd been giving shots for years. I'd put in my hours in the town vet's office after college but I thought it was a big deal to learn what a puppy should weigh at birth. Injections! That was something else again. Even the wild and woolly pig-sticking of the previous summer, which had seemed more an athletic than a medical technique, hadn't prepared me. I was proud of my ability to fill out the certificates in a clear hand while the *vet* gave the vaccinations and other injections. But here I was in class with a syringe in my hand and a dog on the table in front of me and I had to administer a shot.

It's a peculiar sensation to have to do something that you've imagined so many times that it's become routine in your mind

but totally foreign to your body. Anybody can easily imagine
how to give a shot. You just jab the needle in and push, right?
But when the needle is in your hand and the warm flesh is
waiting, courage fails. You think that maybe there's some essential trick to it, some twist or feint that has, for all these
years, escaped you. The skin seems suddenly very thick and
resistant, full of nerves and blood. It's as if real life has become
a cartoon.

The class was anesthesiology. It was an elective and an
exciting one because the labs had lots of direct work with
animals. On that particular day we were comparing the effects
of varying anesthetics. We were going to try Valium and then
ketamine, observe the animals' reactions and see how long it
took them to recover from certain specified dosages. Good
heavens, I thought, heart racing, needle in hand, can't we just
put a pill under their tongues? But no, this was to be the
moment of truth.

We had filled our syringes. The professor told us to make
the injection. It seemed to me that everyone in the class moved
in one fluid motion and completed their injections. I turned
to my partner, my friend Lesley, and whispered very softly,
"Lesley, how do you give a shot?" Seconds later I realized I
had made a terrible mistake. Lesley was not a paragon of tact.
In what seemed to me to be her loudest voice she began a
series of instructions that would have done justice to a drill-
master. "Well, you begin by making a tent of the skin by
pinching it with your fingers like this. . . . You don't want to
go through both layers of skin and shoot the stuff into the air,
do you?" Every face in the lab turned toward me and my face
got redder with Lesley's every word. I couldn't concentrate
on what she was saying. I was certain every other student
thought me a fool and that my inexperience would be the talk
of the campus. But somehow I muddled through and added
yet one more vital technique to my repertoire.

That anesthesiology course provided moments of high
drama. One day we were practicing administering anesthetics

to horses. We were supposed to inject the anesthetic into the neck vein, but you have to be very careful when you do this to a horse. Aside from the obvious cautions incumbent on someone sticking a needle into a large animal, there's an additional potential for trouble: if you stick too deeply you can hit an artery instead of a vein. Then whatever you're injecting travels directly to the brain instead of to the heart. Depending on what you're injecting, that kind of a mistake can kill a horse instantly.

We had had lectures on horse injections and were well aware of how careful we had to be. We knew that once we'd inserted the needle we had to pull back on the plunger a bit. If the blood was bright red, or if it was really spurting under great pressure, it was probably coming from an artery and we would have to withdraw the needle and try again for a vein.

At last the day came for the hands-on work. We gathered excitedly in the fenced-in area beside the large-animal barn. The first student was about to inject an anesthetic into the horse's jugular vein. He was moving quickly and we'll never know if he was trying to convey an impression of expertise or if he was simply forgetful on this, his first, time out. At any rate, he injected the horse quickly and surely like a pro and stood back calmly, the picture of confidence. Then all hell broke loose. The horse's whole body quivered, then his head flew up, then buckled down and he did the first and only equine somersault I've ever seen. The class stood back wide-eyed as the professor got the horse back under control. We all knew instantly what had happened. Had the dosage been larger or of a different drug, the horse could have died on the spot. It was a scary but unforgettable lesson. I'd venture to say that no one in that particular anesthesiology lab ever neglected to carefully monitor their equine injections.

Our anesthesiology professor was an attractive man who was the soul of calm. Nothing ruffled him. In fact perhaps it was his serenity that attracted him to anesthetic work in the first place. I suspected he entertained fantasies of anesthetizing the entire class and perhaps, at his most wanton, the entire student body of OSU. But sometimes his unflappability was infuriating, and one day we decided to do our best to make him at least flinch.

We were administering anesthetics via catheters in the horses' neck veins and evaluating the effects. Once the effect of the anesthetic wore off and the horse began to wake up, we would pull out the catheter. It was then that I thought of a possible way to get a rise out of the professor. The ring finger of my right hand is missing the last joint so that it is only as long as my pinky. I wasn't born that way; I sort of lost my finger at an undergraduate party when someone slammed a door on my hand. It was a violent separation, but I don't miss it at all anymore. At any rate, I figured that half a finger might be just the stimulus to make our phlegmatic professor jump.

After I pulled the catheter out of my horse's neck, I wiped my semi-finger lavishly with blood. Then I approached the professor with an assortment of students, holding my bloodied hand in the other and looking as apprehensive as I could. "The horse bit my finger off," I explained, proffering my shortened digit. My hand looked convincingly grotesque. Everyone in the class waited for him to lose his fabled cool. We expected a cry of alarm, an ambulance, a rush to a hospital.

He looked at my bloodied finger for about ten seconds. Then he nodded to another student. "Get her to the clinic and have them fix her up." He then went to the horse he was working on and turned to us with an afterthought. "And if the horse didn't eat the finger, see if you can find it. Maybe they can stitch it back."

Never try to ruffle an anesthesiology professor.

THE EXTERN AND THE ANTIFREEZE

Sophomore year was the year that you could apply to be an "extern." An extern was a student who lived in the clinic and who was on call after midnight when the regular emergency staff went off duty. Only about ten people were chosen and it was considered a desirable job. An extern got good clinical experience and also free rent. In addition they got part-time paying jobs in the pharmacy or at the front desk. The rooms the externs occupied were primitive. They were small and crowded and, because they were in the clinic building, it was like living in an office off the main floor of Grand Central Station. Moreover, they were located right next to the "cafeteria," or food-machine collection, so the externs had to listen to the constant tinkle of coins and the buzz of the microwave. Only a large glass window separated their living quarters from the cafeteria, so students fueling up on fake food could be entertained by the spectacle of externs emerging from their rooms in their pajamas to use the bathroom down the hall. Hardly a private life. Still, they were getting terrific experience and that was far more valuable than the amenities.

In my sophomore year one of the externs was involved in an incident that brought us all up short. After working long hours all day he was on emergency night duty. He had to answer the clinic phones as well as handle any cases that came in. In the wee hours of the morning the phone in his room rang and he roused himself from sleep to take the call. His roommate, wakened by the ringing, heard one side of the conversation: "Uh huh. Uh huh. Uh huh... Give him some milk and call in the morning."

The next morning the roommate asked why the extern had told the pet owner to give his dog milk. It's an odd recommendation because milk usually causes diarrhea in dogs. A look of profound dismay covered the extern's face. "Did I really *say* that? Oh God! I've got to call those people immediately. . . ."

That late-night call had been about a common problem—antifreeze poisoning. A dog had licked some antifreeze off a garage floor. Antifreeze can be terribly dangerous to pets, dogs, in particular, because it tastes sweet and dogs, who are indiscriminate eaters, like its flavor. If someone spills it on the street or on a driveway or garage floor and a dog comes across it, he'll be very likely to lick it up as if it were beef broth. That's just what this particular dog had done. His owners called the clinic when they noticed the symptoms: the dog was wobbly and very lethargic. Dogs who've ingested anti-freeze are hard to save. The chemicals in the antifreeze bind up in the poisoned dog's kidneys and form damaging crystals. You have to flush the poison out of their systems with alcohol or vodka, put them on intravenous fluids and monitor them in an intensive-care unit. It's a life-threatening emergency.

When the call came in to the extern, he was so exhausted, sleeping so deeply that he never fully wakened. His recom-mendation to give the dog milk came completely out of left field. I don't know if he reached the dog owners in time or if the animal was saved, but the story made a vivid impression on us all. We were all used to staying up late. We were used to gunning long hours. But we always eventually caught up on our sleep and were none the worse for it. Our goal was to get through a test and the worst that could happen was that we would be so tired we wouldn't perform well. Now a new dimension was added to our lives: direct responsibility for the lives of the animals under our care. This was an obligation that went far beyond grades and our first experience with the emotional demands of our profession.

NEW HAMPSHIRE SUMMER

MY FIRST SPAY

I had never been to New Hampshire before and my trip along its winding hilly roads was a revelation. Geology took on new meaning as, leaving the flat plains of Ohio and coming into the eastern mountains, I could imagine the gigantic shifts and shrugs of nature that had produced the terrain. It was a land of views and valleys and Dr. Allen's practice fit right in with the picture-postcard scenery. It was just as Lesley had described it when she told me about the job. Dr. Allen's house was a sprawling white clapboard building—it looked like a mansion to me—and the practice was established in one of the wings.

It was the summer after my sophomore year. Everyone had scattered to work for money or experience. I'd landed a job as a preceptor with Dr. Allen. Lesley had worked for him in the past and she had recommended me for the job. In exchange for room and board with his family, I'd do everything I could to assist Dr. Allen in his practice. If I'd been asked to write the tried-and-true composition, "What I Did Last Summer," the most memorable things I'd have to report were taking up running, performing my first spay, and pulling porcupine quills.

Dr. Allen and his family were running fanatics. Everyone, including his wife and four children, ran up and down the

72

hilly roads of backwoods New Hampshire and before long I'd joined them. We called ourselves the "Plymouth Animal Hospital Turtles."

After a few weeks in New Hampshire I fell into a pleasant routine. I worked in the kennels in the early morning and in the afternoon I ran the heartworm tests and fecal tests and handled the crematorium, which was a dreaded job and it took me a long time to get used to it. Every time I had to put a dog or a cat into the crematorium, I couldn't help but think of their owners and how I would feel if this was happening to my pet. I had a hard struggle to convince myself that it was part of the whole cycle of life, birth and death. I spent the shank of the day with Dr. Allen, assisting him with cases, and in the evening for an hour or two I'd go with him on farm calls. We'd leave at about 7 or 8 P.M. and get home at about 10 P.M. Then the running started. Everyone suited up and hit the roads. At 11 or 11:30 P.M., freshly showered and exhausted, we'd all finally sit down to dinner.

It didn't take long for me to put Dr. Allen on a pedestal. It was an occupational hazard for vet students—roughly equivalent of transference to your shrink.

There was something else about Dr. Allen that was special. He seemed to have managed to combine his work with a happy domestic life. Because his practice was at home he was able to spend more than the usual amount of time with his wife and children. They in turn were able to share in the trials and tribulations of life as a country vet. Long work hours were understood but they seemed less onerous when the kids could stop by for a while to help sort office supplies or walk a patient. The balance of work and family that I saw in New Hampshire crystallized a dilemma for me—one that I'd been only vaguely conscious of for my first two years of vet school.

As a vet student I couldn't help but notice that vets, like MD's, can face strains in their personal lives that are generic to their careers. I suppose it has to do partly with the punishing hours. In just the previous year of school, as I struggled through my endocrine course, I'd had a taste of this as my time spent with Dave was severely curtailed. But he was a student, too, and was sympathetic to the demands on my time. But what, I thought sometimes, if he *weren't* a student? I didn't know what the future held for Dave and me, but I'd been watching other couples in school. There were plenty of vet students married to people outside the profession who were working in other fields and couldn't understand the long hours. In fact, according to school gossip, a few of those marriages were already on shaky ground.

When you finished school, the demands on your time were not lessened. On the contrary, a vet who eventually sets up a practice is really a small businessman with all the worries and headaches of any entrepreneur. But he doesn't close his doors at 5 P.M.; he sometimes works all night with emergency cases.

It seemed to me, watching Dr. Allen, that he'd managed to arrange the best of both worlds. But watching him forced me to acknowledge for the first time that it might not be so easy for me. There was no doubt in my mind what I one day wanted from life: a veterinary practice, a husband and children. But now the seeds of doubt were being planted. Was this a practical goal? Even a possible goal? It was something I would think about for the next few years.

I wanted to be just like Dr. Allen, to handle cases with his precision and sense of caring. I was an eager audience for everything he did. After two years in school, I knew enough to be of some help. But of course I hadn't had much hands-on experience, so many of the things I did were new to me. It's one thing to have a lecture on panleukopenia in a kitten, which is similar to parvo in a dog; it's quite another to have a sick kitten in front of you who looks like she has panleukopenia and an owner waiting for a diagnosis.

In some ways being a vet student is like being an adolescent. You feel you're ready to do much more than you're allowed to do. You're impatient to get on with it. But you're secretly frightened of your ignorance. Going from school to practical situations like summer preceptorships was an excellent remedy. You'd spend nine months eager to get your hands on an animal and three months terrified that you were doing something wrong to the animal you had your hands on. That summer in Plymouth marked the exact middle of vet school education and also the most intense conflict between my confidence and my doubts.

What I most enjoyed was assisting at surgery. In my pre-vet school experience with the town vet he'd performed surgeries during the day and we'd handled mostly outpatient cases in the evening. People would bring their pets in for vaccinations and diarrhea and abscesses and other minor problems. At the time the experience was wonderful for me, but it was limited due to my schedule. In New Hampshire, I was working all day so I was able to observe real live operations. Fall would bring my surgery course and it would be one of the most important in my junior year.

One day we found a "drop-off dog" waiting on the front steps. Drop-off pets are abandoned animals. Some people simply tire of their pets or are financially or physically unable to care for them or find that the animal has a behavioral problem that, most commonly, the owner is responsible for creating and can't correct. So instead of taking the unwanted pet to an animal shelter, they drop them off at a vet's office, assuming the vet will both take care of it and find it a good home. Of course most vets don't have facilities to care for such dogs, especially if they have a busy practice and their kennel is full of dogs recovering or about to be operated on. Still, most vets will try to do the best they can for the drop-offs. This particular orphan was a cute terrier/beagle cross. She looked to be just a few years old and she was friendly and gentle—a likely candidate for adoption.

There is still some controversy today about the best time to spay a female dog. Some vets recommend that you allow the dog to go through one heat; however, most agree that it's best to spay the dog before it's ever come into heat. But there's no argument at all about leaving a dog unspayed. Unless you are a serious breeder and have plans to breed a bitch, she will most likely be healthier and live longer if she's spayed. The incidence of mammary gland tumors (or cancer) in unspayed dogs is very high and 50 percent of such cases are malignant. Intact bitches are equally threatened by uterine infection, otherwise known as pyometra. We figured that our little drop-off hadn't been spayed and I realized that this could be an opportunity for me to do my first spay and at the same time increase her chances of being adopted and living a long, healthy life.

Dr. Allen agreed to let me operate, and early that evening, after office hours, I got the little dog onto the table in the back surgery room. Under Dr. Allen's watchful eyes I administered the preanesthetic into the muscle. As I was setting up the equipment, there was a knock at the door. It was Dr. Allen's wife. She poked her head into the room and said hello. In retrospect, I suppose I should have been immediately suspicious of her amused smile. I continued to fiddle with the equipment, setting up the catheter, drawing up the short-acting anesthetic in the syringe, setting up the endotracheal tube and the anesthetic machine. Once I had everything ready to go, Dr. Allen patted me on the back and said, "Well, Sally, good luck. We're going out to dinner." And with that casual farewell I was alone with a tranquilized dog and a pile of cold instruments.

The spay didn't worry me. I felt pretty confident I would do a creditable job. But as to getting the dog under the anesthetic, that was something else. She was dopey and it was time to put the short-acting anesthetic into the vein on the front of her leg. I'd watched it done a hundred times. But now, suddenly, it seemed the dog's leg was composed of only bone, muscle and fur—not a vein in sight. And the short-acting barbituate I was using had to be injected right into the vein. If you missed and got it into the surrounding tissue it could cause what's known as a "slough" and a few days or even weeks after surgery the animal would begin to slough the skin around the injection site.

Finding a vein is not always easy. You have to insert the needle and then, when you think you're in the vein, slightly withdraw it, keeping negative pressure on the syringe. Only when you get what's called a good "backflush," or flow of blood, do you know that you've hit the vein. Sometimes you can nick the vein in one attempt and it will bleed into the surrounding tissue, forming a hematoma. Then when you make another try, you can see blood in your syringe but it's not from the vein, it's just what's bled out on your failed effort. You can find yourself waiting in vain for a dog to get dopey.

Finally I hit the vein, got the dog anesthetized enough to place a tube down her trachea and connected her to the anesthetic machine. I was on my way. The door opened again and in walked two of Dr. Allen's four children. A boy and a girl, both high school students, they'd come to watch my first surgery. With the unerring instinct of the young, they sensed that what was going on in surgery was far more interesting than anything happening on TV that evening. At first I was pleased to have the company and an audience, until they began a running commentary: "Gee, that sure was a nice dog. Oh well..."

Ignoring the peanut gallery, I calmly made the incision and prepared to search for the ovary. Although a spay is common, it's major abdominal surgery. The first step is finding the ovaries quickly. A bitch's reproductive tract is shaped like an elongated "Y." The two ovaries are located at the top tips. The two tubes leading from the ovaries are called the uterine horns and they are where the puppies develop. In effect, the bitch has two long uteruses. The base of the "Y" is the cervix. In the course of a spay you need to remove the ovaries and the two uterine horns by making a cut at the top of the cervix and by tying off the ovarian vessels.

Speed is a factor in successful surgery. The faster you can get in and get out, the less chance of complications arising from anesthetic or infection. I wanted to find this dog's ovaries quickly. Because the dog is on its back and the ovaries are located near the spine, you usually have to do some poking around before you find them. Sometimes you don't find them at all. Occasionally—rarely, really—you'll have a herma-phrodite dog—one with both male and female sex organs. Much more common is the "second spay" syndrome where someone brings in a dog to be spayed but once you get in you find it's already been spayed. This happens occasionally with stray dogs that have been adopted.

I was ready to begin my ovarian search under the watchful eyes of Dr. Allen's kids. I was prepared to impress them and maybe even teach them something along the way. "I'm now going to locate the ovary," I announced. "Sally, why don't you try the spay hook?" the girl replied. In an instant, the evening fell into place. These were not innocent kids. They knew more about surgery than *I* did. They'd probably been watching their father do spays for half their lives. They'd probably been watching preceptors fumble their way through spays for nearly as long. At first I was embarrassed but then grateful. They'd be my safety net.

I picked up the spay hook, a long instrument with a hook at the end that you can use to pull out the uterine horn. (Now that I'm more experienced I use only my hands because I can find the uterine horns more quickly by touch—they feel like ropes while the intestines feel flatter and softer.) I was sweating from the July heat and tension. I had to keep looking up to the ceiling so the sweat would run behind my ears and not into my incision. When I had gathered my courage, I reached down with the spay hook and in a few seconds pulled out something that I hoped against hope had something to do with reproduction. What luck! I got the uterine horn first try. I looked up in triumph at my audience. They glanced at one another, obviously impressed.

The next difficult aspect of a spay is tying off the ovarian stump. You have to be scrupulous about making your tie. You have to tie off the stump securely enough so it won't continue to bleed, as the vessels branch off the aorta and, if not tied correctly, the pet may bleed to death. If the dog is fat, you have to be careful you don't let excess fat tissue get tied up with the stump, thereby minimizing the pressure of your knot on the vessels. I completed that part of the surgery without a hitch and by then didn't expect any cheers from the peanut gallery.

By the time I sutured that dog and removed the tracheal tube, I was exhausted, and sweat-drenched. Still, when the little dog coughed and began to regain some color, I was the happiest person in New Hampshire. It's hard to describe what a thrill it is to work on an animal, hold its organs in your hands, sew it back up and have it bounce back the next day wagging its tail and ready to chase squirrels. Few subsequent surgeries gave me the pleasure of that first spay. And as I cleaned up the table, the two experts finally broke down and told me I'd done a great job. I felt like I'd just won an Academy Award.

The next day when I came into the reception room of the office I saw a new display had appeared on the bulletin board. There was a sign on the top of the board—"Sally's First Spay"—and beneath it were Polaroid photos of me. There I was fishing for the uterine horns. There I was sweating as I tied off the ovarian stump. And finally there I was, grinning idiotically, pulling the tube from the dog's throat. I felt like a bride getting the wedding prints a month after the event. Had this really happened? When did they take all these photos? I'd been so engrossed I never heard the shutter snapping. And those kids were as experienced as professional wedding photographers. I suppose every preceptor left New Hampshire with a collection of "first surgery" snaps. I didn't care if it was routine for them; I was so happy to have those photos, and even now I enjoy taking them out and looking at them and remembering the excitement and anxiety of that first spay.

The little dog, the heroine of the story really, recovered

beautifully. When I visited her the next morning she was full of pep and held no grudges. Within a week a client who'd lost a dog was happy to take her home and I hope today finds her still chasing chipmunks in the lush New Hampshire woods.

PORCUPINES AND A MOOSE

We all know that nature has a way of making the best food hard to get. Oysters, artichoke hearts and caviar all take some work. Dogs, it seems, have arrived at this conclusion on their own. Whether because of their superior intelligence or their vast experience unlidding garbage cans, we'll never know, but they recognize that the most succulent tidbits take the most effort. And one thing they're certain of—porcupine makes great eating. I'm sure that when they lie around on dusty New Hampshire roads in the afternoon, they dream of curling their tongues around a succulent porcupine. The first thing a dog new to New England hears after he sniffs his way around the local talent is that there's no finer eating. The fact that the dog passing on the news has never been nearer to a porcupine belly than an eight-inch quill is never disclosed.

The first porcupine victim I'd ever seen was a small dog— a beagle mix—who was brought in with a mouth full of quills. Often a dog will just sniff around a porcupine wondering why the local curs extoll its meat when it doesn't seem to have any. These dogs usually wind up with multiple quills implanted in their gums and hard palate. But my first case was one of the most extreme I've ever seen. He must have been right off the boat because he'd obviously trotted up to a porcupine as if it were a discarded bologna sandwich and taken a giant bite. He was in terrible shape when he got to us with some dozens of quills lodged in his mouth and face. He couldn't even close his jaws and was surely in agony, to say nothing of how embarrassed he must have been at branding himself a rube.

Porcupine quills have a sort of barb at the tip so you can't just pull them out cleanly. They hurt as much coming out as going in, perhaps more, so our first priority was to sedate the dog. In order to remove a quill, you take a hemostat—the surgical instrument that became popular in the 1960s as a holder for joints—grab the quill and yank. Sometimes you'll be lucky and get it all out on the first pull. Other times the quill will break. Then you have to dig to get out as much of the remaining quill as you can because if a piece is left in it can form an abscess and infection. However, in some cases the quill is buried so deeply you leave it alone in hopes that it will eventually dissolve or work its way out.

We worked for an hour on that poor beagle and it was one of those occasions that makes you grateful for the effectiveness of modern anesthetics. Without anesthesia, the pain would surely overshadow the immediate problem of getting the quills out. And you'd run the risk of getting bitten every time you reached back into the throat with the hemostat.

We finally had the beagle almost completely de-quilled. There were still a few black specks indicating fragments in his face but we hoped they'd ultimately work their way out. We kept the beagle overnight and the next day he was in fine shape. He came back in about a week for a checkup as blithely oblivious as if the encounter had never happened. No doubt he's right now advising a new dog that he hasn't *eaten* till he's chomped down on a porcupine. There should be a rule that such a dog must wear a canine version of the scarlet letter— a porcupine quill dangling from the collar—to alert unwary dogs to the dangers of high living.

Dogs aren't the only ones who have run-ins with porcupines. We had a horse who came in with a leg full of quills. He must have been walking unwarily past a porcupine that panicked and unleased some lateral force. We sedated the horse and spent about a half hour with our hemostats pulling quills. The horse recovered nicely and is probably the sort of good equine citizen who warns his stable mates about the dangers of those small, sharp animals.

One of the interesting aspects of working with unusual animals is that you are forced to use your ingenuity to adapt techniques and equipment to a new situation. The summer I was in New Hampshire, one of my biggest challenges was a moose with a broken leg.

One especially warm afternoon we got a call from someone in the forest service. They had come across a moose in trouble. At that time the closest I'd come to a moose was a head mounted on a wall. I had seen a whole one once at a zoo when I was a child and remembered vaguely that it was about the most unshapely animal I'd ever seen with a lot of superfluous parts. Given what I knew of their construction, it was hard to imagine how I would be able to tell that something was wrong with a moose, unless his head was missing, in which case I wasn't optimistic about the prognosis.

When the moose arrived it shattered all my moose stereotypes. It was shaggy and shy and looked a lot like Bullwinkle. As it was a young moose, it hadn't yet reached the skyscraper proportions of the adult, which can tower over six feet at the shoulder and weigh as much as a Volkswagen. It did seem to have a lot of excess, somehow inappropriate parts that made it look like a first rough sketch for a deer. And it immediately endeared itself to me because it was an easy diagnosis. It was obvious at first glance what was wrong: he had a broken leg. Perhaps it was the pain, perhaps fear, but this moose was as cool and composed as his wall-mounted brethren. Nonetheless, the ranger warned us that a moose crossed can be formidable.

First we had to determine if it was a clean break or a ragged one and if there were multiple pieces of bone that had broken off. We had to X-ray the leg. Which meant we had to coax his bulk through the human-sized doorframe and into the tiny X-ray room and then hold him still while we used expensive and delicate machinery in the vicinity of his only method of self-defense: his hoofs and shovel-like horns.

As I helped Dr. Allen maneuver the moose through the

hospital—too engrossed in our problem to realize how funny we looked—I thought back to the high-strung thoroughbred horse with the same problem that we had X-rayed back at school the previous year. But the horse was violent and, even though he was tranquilized and restrained with a twitch, no one could hold him still enough to get the work done. I had volunteered to go into the padded X-ray room and help out when a number of other students, no doubt more experienced and wiser than I, had refused. We had to hold the horse's leg just so, so that the angle of the X ray would be useful. To do this we had to maneuver the horse so that he bent his leg and, in effect, stood on his toe. We did this by resting the front of his hoof in a grooved block of wood to keep the foreleg at the correct angle. Once we got the leg into position, we had to move our own hands so we wouldn't be exposed to the X rays. After numerous fruitless tries, the horse got disgusted with this amateur ballet step and decided to show us a *grand jeté*. He soared into the air, smack into the X-ray machine. The X-ray machine was suspended from a track on the ceiling. The impact sent it sliding crazily along the track until it hit the far wall. I lost my grip on the horse after I was hauled into the air and, following the X-ray machine, I flew into the wall and slid into a heap on the floor. I was stunned but still alert enough to appreciate the death of the X-ray machine as it slammed into the wall and exploded in a fireworks finale. It was a memorable afternoon, yielding no X ray and costing one $10,000 machine.

I thought it prudent to keep this story to myself as we at last got our moose into the X-ray room. Dr. Allen didn't have such expensive equipment but he also didn't have an endowment so I kept my checkered past a secret. But as it turned out, though we had to do a lot of maneuvering, we had a reasonable picture within an hour. The moose had a clean break in his right foreleg. We'd have to put a cast on him and keep him off the leg for at least six weeks. It was important to keep the moose as motionless as possible while his leg healed or else the bones might not heal together properly and hamper his future mobility.

The most suitable spot for creating the moose cast was the front lawn of the practice, as it provided space and light and lots of room to spread out both moose and plaster. Most every car in Plymouth, New Hampshire, stopped or at least slowed down to rubberneck. I kept imagining the skepticism that would greet dinner-table conversation that night whenever a witness claimed that he'd seen a moose getting a leg casted on a lawn that afternoon. Even a sworn teetotaler would have a rough go with that one. The only one, in fact, unmoved by the situation was the moose himself, who was the soul of dignity throughout.

Getting the cast on was one thing, but keeping him off his feet *after* the cast was on required some improvising. We got the moose into Dr. Allen's barn and rigged up a sort of sling from the sides of neighboring stalls so that he wouldn't be putting any weight on his leg. We strung fresh leaves and grass from a rope in front of his nose so that he could nibble at will. For the next few weeks that moose was king of the stable. He reigned with great aplomb and even permitted interviews by the press as a local media sensation. Celebrity didn't tarnish his good nature and we all began to recognize that his absurd exterior housed a truly noble soul. We kept careful watch over him and fed him damp leaves picked from the trees surrounding the practice and any greenery we could find that would tempt his appetite. I enjoyed visiting him in the cool of the New England morning with some fresh greens and I would stand stroking his horns talking to him, trying to convince him that soon he would be back among his own with wet feet and all the comforts of home.

A couple of weeks went by and I was convinced our moose was doing well. But one sad day we realized he was declining—even the tastiest green morsels went untouched. Within a few days he was dead. We'll never know if he died from complications connected to his cast or his captivity or from

some moose disease he'd contracted before he found his way
to Dr. Allen's. Perhaps he simply missed standing in water
and gazing out across the New Hampshire lakes to far mountains, dreaming his moose dreams.

PLUM ISLAND

When my friend Lesley called to invite me to Plum Island,
I knew that it was a center for exotic diseases of large animals
but I didn't even know where it was. I had gotten permission
from Dr. Allen to take an extended weekend to visit Lesley
and then to go on to New York City to see the Animal Medical
Center. The whole weekend certainly had the ring of educational improvement to it.

Plum Island is shaped like a eight-hundred-acre pork chop
floating across Long Island Sound to Connecticut. Separated
from the north fork of Long Island by a few miles of turbulent
waters known as Plum Gut, it is extremely isolated. Sailors
braving the violent currents of the Gut on their way to Connecticut and northern sailing grounds can see the island off to
their right as they head north but indeed there's not much to
see. Plum Island is relatively flat and sandy, and covered with
scrub pine. It hasn't much attraction for anyone but the government, which owns the island and has given it over, all eight
hundred acres, to the Plum Island Animal Disease Center, a
government facility established in 1954 to serve as a laboratory
for studying foreign, also known as "exotic," animal diseases.
Given the danger of the communicable diseases studied, it has
the ideal geography. It's reached only by regular ferry from
the mainland, but only the employees of the center or autho-
rized personnel can board that ferry. To be allowed to visit
with Lesley, I had had to have a special clearance that required
me to swear that I wouldn't treat or encounter large animals
for a two-week duration after my visit to the island. I had
worked this out in advance with Dr. Allen, who had agreed

that I would skip the large-animal calls in the evening for two weeks after my Plum Island visit.

While at first this caution may seem excessive, when you realize that diseases like foot-and-mouth disease, which is unknown in this country, can kill millions of cattle and could ricochet across the country causing an increase of as much as 50 percent in meat prices, it is more than justified. Plum Island is really our country's first line of defense against invasion by foreign diseases. Due to the studies done there, vets from all over the U.S. visit Plum Island to learn to recognize diseases that are nonexistent here. In addition to research and education, the personnel at Plum Island are available to diagnose any suspicious diseases that veterinarians across the country might discover.

Plum Island personnel also run testing centers in other parts of the nation. For example, livestock that's being imported to the U.S. from a country that has a history of foot-and-mouth disease undergo a routine series of tests. First they are held in their country of origin until the U.S. Department of Agriculture can test them. Animals found entirely free of symptoms are shipped to Fleming Key in Florida, where the Plum Island people run additional tests. Only after the animals pass the Plum Island scrutiny are they certified free of foot-and-mouth and shipped to their American destinations.

After a quiet evening of catching up with Lesley on summer activities, we rode the ferry to Plum Island the next morning from Orient on the north fork of Long Island. I had expected to be most interested in the animals and procedures at the center but I found myself marveling instead at the security system that was geared to contain not armed robbers or rabid animals but germs, viruses and bacteria that could escape the island on a human or animal host and alter the agricultural future of America. High chain-link fences surrounded the facilities. They were intended not only to keep any diseased animals inside but also to keep out any innocent wild animals or straying boats that might find their way to the island. The laboratories themselves have a peculiar system of air control. The air pressure inside is kept lower than that of the outside air. This makes it impossible for any air from the inside to escape to the outside bearing dangerous viruses or other contaminants. Highly sophisticated filtering systems cleanse the air that finally leaves the labs.

Most amazing to me was the shower system that only a mother of preadolescent boys could love. Every time you went into a different lab area, you had to shower. A Plum Island shower is no quick rinse. You have to scrub your entire body with special soaps. You are given little devices designed to perfect the efficiency of your under-the-fingernail scrub. You have to wash your hair. My day at Plum Island included five showers, not counting the one I'd taken that morning civilian-style. One vet told me of a fifteen-shower marathon he had taken one day on Plum Island. If the cleansing action of those showers was cumulative, a summer intern could probably skip bathing of any kind for the year following his internship.

The day that I spent on Plum Island was devoted largely to African swine fever, a disease of pigs unknown in the U.S. at present. First we saw a film on the disease that showed the symptoms of diseased animals and how a vet could recognize the disease. Then we saw the sick pigs, which had been imported from another country, and examined their symptoms. Pigs with African swine fever will have a drop in temperature from a feverish state to around 99 degrees right before they die. After we'd examined the pigs, clinicians killed and autopsied them and we examined the lesions of swine fever.

After our mini-course on swine fever, we jumped into the shower and Lesley took me to visit the lab where she worked. After a tour of the lab and another shower, it was time for lunch. The afternoon was devoted to a few more showers, some lab work and a short tour of other parts of the facility. As I wasn't really interested in working with large animals in the future, Plum Island was more a curiosity to me than anything else. But the six vet students who were there as summer interns seemed to be having a wonderful time as well as an educational experience living on the idyllic north fork of Long Island, riding the ferry to and from work and showering, showering, showering.

The next day one of the Plum Island vet students had business to conduct in New York at the Animal Medical Center and Lesley and I and several others tagged along for the ride. Who could say no to a visit to the most famous animal medical hospital in the country if not the world? Only Angell Memorial in Boston has a comparable reputation. I'd been hearing about the AMC for years. It was a Mecca for vet students because it has the best facilities, the best people and a fantastic caseload. I thought as I'd probably be practicing in the Midwest in the future, I'd grab what might be my only chance to visit the AMC.

We rolled across the Queensborough Bridge early in the morning and suddenly I knew what "rush-hour traffic" meant. The kind I was used to in Ohio meant a row of cars instead of one or two. But this was traffic. This was another world, another culture based on waiting and taking chances. It was a marvelous entry into the city.

When we drove up to the entrance of the AMC on Sixty-second Street near York Avenue, if it hadn't been for the sign on the building I would have been sure my friends were playing a practical joke on me. This humble place *couldn't* be the famous Animal Medical Center. To get to the entrance you drove under the building itself where a small parking lot crouched. The plate-glass entrance doors opened to reveal an old tiled foyer, a bench, a sort of card table with pamphlets on it and a reception desk. Two giant elevator doors filled one wall and behind the reception desk the tile floor became a ramp that led upward to another floor. Everything looked old and shabby. At Ohio State, the veterinary clinic was virtually new. Everything was stainless steel, bright and shiny as a new penny. But the AMC, at least on first impression, was virtually decrepit. I felt like I was peeking behind the machine run by the Wizard of Oz.

Our friend had his meeting at the AMC and we left, glad to be out in the charged air of the city. Until the wee hours of the next morning we explored New York on the veterinary version of a busman's holiday: we saw the Off-Broadway play *P.S. Your Cat Is Dead*, we ate octopus and visited the Museum of Natural History, where we got to see more bones than we'd seen in all our years combined.

JUNIOR YEAR

SURGERY

The beginning of junior year was one of the most exhilarating times of my whole veterinary education. As I returned to Columbus after the New Hampshire summer, even the flat land looked good to me. I was so eager to be back at school, to see my friends again and learn about their summers. I'd also missed Dave and was glad to be back with him, taking up where we'd left off.

This year I would share an apartment with Skid and her friend Shelley. Skid was working at Ohio State and Shelley was a social worker in Columbus so I was the only student in the group. We settled into our town-house apartment with zest. Skid and Shelley did most of the serious decorating and homemaking and I was grateful for their efforts. As far as they were concerned, there was only one blot on our domestic arrangement: Watson. Watson was a New Zealand red rabbit who I'd brought back from New Hampshire with me. He was a warm brown color and looked like a wild rabbit except he had the large ears of domestic. He also had the large appetite of the domestic rabbit and quickly nibbled most of Skid's plants down to nubbins. Skid and Shelley were not thrilled about sharing their apartment with a rabbit but they were gracious about it. They even included him in our quarterly parties.

By the end of our junior year our quarterly theme parties

had become legend. We would pick a theme—a potluck picnic or a toga party or a mad hatter's party—and throw open the doors of our apartment to everyone we knew. At our first mad hatter's party, Skid and Shelley were kind enough to include Watson in the festivities and, wearing the little top hat I'd made for him, with holes for his elegant ears, he hopped off with first prize. But, as the prize was a six-pack of beer and as Watson was on the wagon, some dissidents demanded a recount and the prize was wrested from Watson's disappointed paws.

It didn't take long before Shelley, Skid and I were comfortably into the rhythm of our life together. They'd come to OTS—the veterinary fraternity—parties with me and I'd go to work-related parties with them. Except for the occasional strain of Watson, we were a happy group. But there was another relationship that began in my junior year that was to become just as important to me. And it began in, of all places, surgery lab.

By Christmas of junior year I'd decided that living together is no real test of a relationship. You can always escape to a movie, order out for a meal or call in a maid. If you really want to test the mettle of two people joined as one, I recommend you act as partners for a quarter course in animal surgery. If you finish as friends, it will be despite the fact that you've seen the worst of one another under enormous pressure in situations where your success depends on the skill and stamina of your partner.

For the vet who didn't go on to do postgrad work, surgery class was the main opportunity to learn the techniques you'd be using once you got out into practice. Some large veterinary practices have people who specialize in surgery but most vets do everything—medicine and surgery—themselves. And there's so much to learn! No matter how much experience you've had with animals, you can't imagine what it's like to make an incision or tie off a pumping artery until you've actually done it.

But there were other factors that made surgery exciting and sometimes terrifying. It's your introduction to "performance anxiety." Through freshman and sophomore years you've been depending on your mind to get you through tests and papers. But now, like a dancer or an athlete, you've got to depend on your body. To be a good surgeon, you have to be dexterous. You're not just marking a multiple-choice question; you're slicing through skin, opening organs and mending bones.

In surgery you're not just graded on the final result. An instructor circulates throughout the whole procedure and your every move, your speed and your general progress are monitored. It was a major change of pace for people who'd spent two years with their noses buried in books. For some students, surgery proved a nightmare. The ones who suffered most were the "bookish" students who studied obsessively and had excellent grades. Suddenly they found themselves in an unfamiliar arena, with a different kind of audience and a whole new set of expectations.

There was another aspect to surgery that made it particularly intense. Until we began the course, the competition among students was black and white and simple. You got a higher or a lower grade. Now not only was the competition on a different basis—performance instead of grades—but we could watch one another at work. Within a few weeks of the beginning of surgery we all knew who was naturally deft, who was hopelessly slow, who was a terrible klutz.

Given the intense pressure, it's easy to see that your surgery partner—the person you work with on every operation—is a crucial factor in your own success. My selection of a surgery partner had all the earmarks of a bad marriage. I had chosen a friend, a man, who was funny and relaxed and smart. I thought we'd be an excellent pair and was relieved when he agreed to work with me. But a few days after our betrothal, he decided to postpone his surgery course from the first quarter of the term to the second so he could work with another student. I'd been abandoned, not quite at the altar, but in the church vestibule, and I needed to find a groom pronto. Some-

one told me that a girl named Lorraine had also been dumped
by her intended. I knew Lorraine, but not really well. She
seemed like a nice person—I'd never seen her kick a dog or
incite to riot. But she did have a flaw: she was known as
"Lorraine the Brain." I'm certainly not averse to some stim-
ulating competition but I didn't want to spend the semester
playing Watson to someone's Holmes. On the other hand, I
didn't have much choice.

To my great relief, Lorraine agreed to partner me. Aside
from the ominous significance of her nickname, we had another problem to overcome. During the course you and your
partner are working together on the same animal for every
operation. The surgery tables are adjustable so you can set
them at any height. But when Lorraine and I stood before our
table we realized that no adjustment would satisfy us both.
Lorraine is about five feet tall and I'm almost half a foot taller.
If she could work comfortably, I'd be bent in half. If the table
was set for me, Lorraine had to operate on tiptoes. Finally we
reached a compromise: Lorraine stood on something—a box,
some books, whatever was handy—and we finally saw eye to
eye.

Despite those tenuous beginnings, Lorraine and I, like As-
taire and Rogers or Bob and Ray, had that special, indefinable
chemistry that makes for magic partnerships and, in our opin-
ions at least, we became legends in student surgery history.

Of course legends don't always begin in perfection. So it
was the first day of surgery lab. We had surgery twice a week.
We would first be expected to read up on the surgery we
would be doing, then we would be quizzed and graded on the
procedure. Next we would move to our tables—two people
and one animal per table—and begin. But before we could
do any real work we would have to prep ourselves and the
animal. For an experienced vet, this usually takes about ten
or fifteen minutes. It will give you some idea of our ignorance
to tell you that just to prepare the animal would take us anywhere from one to two hours.

Our first surgery was a spay on a dog. The small animals

we operated on came from the local pounds. They were animals that had been abandoned and, in many cases, they were sick. Some of the dogs had distemper, a common, fatal disease. Sometimes the animals recovered from our surgeries, especially the ones that weren't sick in the first place, and they went back to the pound where we all hoped they finally found homes.

Lorraine and I were so excited about our first surgery we couldn't wait to get our hands on our instruments. This would be my big chance to demonstrate that perfect grades weren't the most important sign of a great vet. I would be swift and sure and even Lorraine would be impressed. We knew we had to prepare our dog first and then scrub up ourselves but we figured we'd be getting down to business in short order. That was before we met our dog.

She had veins of steel or, in a few crucial places, none at all. Once we had administered the preanesthetic we tried to insert the catheter into the vein but we soon became convinced our dog had been victimized by a vampire. All her veins seemed to be collapsed or gone. Every time we thought we saw the thin blue line on the middle of her front leg that indicated a vein, we'd press it and it would immediately disappear. Our initial delicacy gave way to more clumsy attempts to get the catheter into place in the dog's leg that at least *resembled* a vein and finally, after what seemed like countless attempts, we succeeded. We looked up at one another and smiled with the thrill of accomplishment.

We'd been working only a few minutes but we already felt as if we'd spent the entire morning in the big, brightly lit surgery room. But we had made progress—our dog was anesthetized and completely relaxed. I silently apologized to her for the clumsy treatment she'd gotten so far and promised we'd do better from that moment on. We lifted her head, opened her mouth and, with the aid of a flashlight, looked into her throat. A piece of cake, we thought. For once, we were right, or at least lucky. The endotracheal tube went into place without a hitch. When we lifted our heads from our dog we noticed that, despite our start-up problems, we were finished before most of the others. Perhaps I had some natural talent as a surgeon after all. "Lorraine the Brain" might have been used to this exhilaration but I was a virgin. It felt awfully good to find myself doing so well so early on.

It's almost impossible to make people and animals completely sterile but, for the purposes of the operating room, you want to eliminate as much bacteria as you can. The more bacteria floating around, the greater the chance of infection and postoperative problems. In order to maintain as germ-free an environment as possible, you "prep" the animal and then you "prep" yourself.

Lorraine and I returned to our dog in the prep room—a room that was just behind the main surgery room. We clipped her abdomen carefully, letting the fur fall into piles on the floor. As we were the first to begin to clip our dog, the floor was white when we entered. By the time the entire class was finished, the floor would be covered with fur in all colors of the animal rainbow. Once our dog was hairless from her chest to her vulva we moved her to the surgery table in the surgery room and began her sterile scrub. We washed her twice with the Betadine scrub. Then we followed with alcohol. For each scrub you move your gauze pad in a square pattern beginning in the center and moving always toward the outer perimeter, keeping any contamination away from the freshly scrubbed skin. Lorraine and I moved easily through this routine and in a short time our dog was ready for the spay. Now we had to prepare ourselves.

"Sterile prep," or scrubbing up, involved the most fastidious hand-washing routine imaginable that, with practice, becomes quick and simple but especially that first time is an endless, tedious ritual. Before you begin to do the actual scrubbing you put on your cap and mask. If, like Lorraine and me, you have long hair, it takes forever to tuck every single strand under the white edge of your cap. We were later to discover that if you pinch the mask where it rests above the bridge of your nose, it will stay in place more readily. I also learned, weeks later, that chewing gum isn't the best policy. Once, during a particularly long procedure, I was chewing merrily away when the gum slipped out of my mouth and into my mask. Of course I couldn't break sterile technique to get the gum out so I worked for hours with a cold lump of Wrigley's Spearmint resting next to my chin.

When we were finally wearing our caps and masks, we were ready to scrub up. Using an antiseptic such as Betadine you begin by washing your fingers. Imagine that each finger has four surfaces—top, bottom, and two sides. When you scrub up, you rub each surface of each finger ten times: top of the finger ten times, bottom of the finger ten times, side of the finger ten times and so on. That means forty passes to each finger, two hundred passes per hand, four hundred passes and your fingers are done and you're ready to move on to your palms. After a few hundred rubs on the front and then the back of your hands, you slowly make your way up your wrists and finally your forearms. It's a great moment when you finally get within striking distance of your elbows.

All this rubbing takes its toll. I never minded scrubbing in the winter but in the summer I hated it because I knew I was washing off my hard-earned tan. Each of the hundreds of passes across my skin removed more of my golden glow and replaced it with an orange stain. Our class took surgery in three groups over three different quarters and you could have picked all the surgery students out of a class lineup because they were the ones with orange-tinged fingers. Eventually we realized that Phisohex didn't stain the way Betadine did and most of us switched. In the summer you recognized Phisohex fans because they looked like they were wearing pale rubber gloves while the Betadine devotees looked like they were sporting an "instant tan."

Once you were up to your elbows in antiseptic, you had to rinse and you had to do it carefully or you would just be spreading all the bacteria around rather than washing it off. It was at this point in the procedure that you assumed the praying mantis posture of the half-scrubbed surgeon. With both arms extended, elbows bent and palms facing you, you would begin by putting your hands under the stream of water from the high faucet with your fingers pointing upward. Once your fingertips were rinsed, you'd move your arms forward and up so your elbows would be the last rinsed. All this scrubbing and rinsing in the peculiar posture of a surgeon took its toll: the first few weeks of junior year my arms ached constantly. Eventually my muscles got into condition for surgery but in the beginning every time I opened a window or reached for a book on a high shelf I felt the twinge in my arms.

Finally, we were scrubbed and rinsed and it was time to find someone to gown us. Despite your thousand-rub scrub, your hands are clean but not sterile, and the idea is to keep them from touching the outside of the sterile gown. So you pick up the gown from the inside and push your arms into, but not through, the sleeves. Then someone ties the gown behind you. At last, both Lorraine and I looked like surgeons.

We were ready for what is called a "closed-glove technique." This means getting a pair of surgical gloves on your hands without touching the sterile outside of them. The gloves are half inside out and you have to slip your fingers in, one hand at a time, always keeping the sterile from the unsterile. The challenge ranks with trying to put on pantyhose before your nail polish has dried and it's a maneuver I've noticed female vet students take to more readily than males.

When Lorraine and I returned to our dog, "suited up," we felt like new women, certainly not the two girls who'd begun scrubbing the tops of their fingers fifteen minutes ago. Nonetheless we felt like impostors in our blue gowns and sterile gloves. It would be a few weeks before we became unconscious of our surgical outfits and longer before we could put them on in less than a quarter of an hour.

As the students trickled back to the operating room, I noticed that everyone was looking a bit sheepish, though our masks, thankfully, hid any self-conscious grins. Our dog, with her bright orange belly, was looking far more relaxed than either of us and we took heart from her unwitting display of confidence.

Beside the operating table is another, smaller table and on it were our surgery packs. Inside each one were our sterile instruments and our drapes, really like large blue towels. In order to keep the working area as sterile as possible, you cover the animal with drapes, one over the front, one over the back and one on each side, and you use towel clamps to attach them gently to the skin. Then you take a large drape that has a slit cut in it and cover the whole table. You center the slit on the area you're working on and through it you have access to the animal. Once the animal is draped, you could never tell what it is and, if it weren't for the anesthesia and oxygen machines at each of the fifteen tables, you'd think the room was filled with pairs of people bending over piles of laundry with the same rectangular orange stains.

Surgery class began at 1 P.M. and ended at 5. Of course, the five o'clock finish was a formality. You had to stay until you were finished with the operation. And then you had to stop the anesthetic and wait until the animal could swallow so that you could pull the endotracheal tube. As our weeks of surgery continued into the winter and we became more experienced, Lorraine and I realized that the quicker the animal was off the anesthetic, the less the chance of problems due to the toll anesthesia takes on the body. And, of course, the sooner we'd get to leave. So we began experimenting with ways of getting our animals to come to more quickly. Many students didn't realize that if you just let the animal wake up on its own, it could take hours. But if you stimulate the patient by flipping it gently from one side to the other, both sides of the lungs will aerate and it will be awake much more quickly. But on that first surgery we still had a lot to

learn. It was about four o'clock and we were finally ready
to cut. If we continued at this rate, I figured it would take
us about three years to complete the one-quarter surgery
course. The only thing that made me feel better was that
there were students who were even slower. As our stomachs
growled, we realized that on surgery days we'd have to have
a very big lunch.

So finally, with Lorraine poised on her stack of books, we
selected the proper instruments from our surgery packs and
prepared to make that first cut. Suddenly I saw a movement
at the door to the operating room. There was a small window
in the door and I could see Dave peering through the window
and waving to me. Being a year ahead of me, he had probably
forgotten that your first surgery class is endless. He certainly
looked amazed to see that we hadn't even begun yet. I waved
to him and smiling, I scratched my nose. His expression
changed completely. He rolled his eyes and shook his head.
He pushed the door open a crack—no one who's not scrubbed
up is allowed in the operating room—and said, "Sally, you
broke sterile technique." As all the white heads in the room
swiveled toward me, I remembered my nose. I could still feel
a little tingle on the tip of it. I had scratched my unsterile
nose with my sterile surgery gloves. I was sure that everyone
was grinning beneath their masks as I returned to the scrub
room to repeat the endless process. Lorraine swore she wasn't
laughing, but I'm sure I saw her mask vibrating.

Despite all our false starts our first surgery was a success.
The next day, as we ran into the recovery room to check our
patient, I began to appreciate an interesting phenomenon about
our feelings toward our animals. As surgical students our ob-
jectives were sometimes different from our professors'. While
we were graded on the precision and skill of a procedure, we
were often more concerned with its outcome. We wanted our
animals to live. A healthy patient was tangible proof of our
skill as surgeons. This didn't diminish our concern for grades:
we were always competitive about that. Still, an "A" on the

procedure was not much consolation on those occasions when you arrived early in the morning to find your animal dead in its cage. Often, before you even found the animal, someone would be eager to give you the bad news. The day after a surgery, students combed the recovery cage area first thing in the morning and every newcomer was greeted with the news of the results. If someone's animal died, the obit spread like wildfire and you felt it was a personal stigma. In the worst cases you lost an animal—usually a dog—that you really cared about. In fact it was unrealistic to expect your patients to survive every procedure; most of the animals we operated on were sick to begin with and some had almost no hope of a good prognosis.

Lorraine and I had extremely good luck with our patients and our postop survival rate was very respectable. I think it was largely due to the fact that we managed to pick animals that were fairly healthy, but we preferred to believe it was due to our skill and there must have been some nugget of truth in that. We were always especially thrilled to find our patients in good shape because our approach to surgical procedures was much more relaxed and commonsensical than that of many of our fellow students. We relied on our instincts as well as on the books and we spent a certain amount of time laughing and playing practical jokes. Many of the other students thought we were goofing off. We were pleased to have live, recovering animals to vindicate us.

But all these things we learned as time went on. After that first spay we wanted only to find our little dog well and on her way to recovery. So that morning when we rushed into the recovery room and up to her cage, our hearts were in our mouths. But sure enough, that little dog scrambled to her feet and her whole body wiggled with pleasure at our company. It was hard to believe that just the day before we'd been working inside her body with scalpels and sutures. It was a thrilling morning for both Lorraine and me—one I'll certainly never forget.

101

DEM BONES, DEM BONES...

I don't believe I was ever destined to be the fastest surgeon around but I was determined to be the most fastidious. I wanted all my incisions to be the straightest and my stitches to look like the seams on a major-league baseball. Sometimes I drove Lorraine crazy when I insisted we take out stitches I didn't think were precise enough. If the stitches were crooked or too tight, puckering the skin, I would insist that we remove them and then resuture the incision. Of course if you just sutured it up all over again, it could look even worse because of the new holes, so I would be sure that we used those holes we'd already made, unless it was essential to add some new ones. Lorraine sometimes claimed that I used a tiny ruler to get those seams just right but that's an exaggeration.

But there was a rationale to my compulsiveness. For most pet owners the stitches are the emblem of the surgeon's skill. When their pet comes home they examine what they can see of the incision and their opinion of the skill of the surgeon will be made on the basis of what's before their eyes. No matter that the surgeon has done an extraordinary job on their pet's interior, if the stitches look like a bunny's path across a meadow, it will be hard to believe the inside looks much better.

So I admit my main reason for priding myself on my sutures was cosmetic. Nonetheless, it's that sort of compulsiveness that makes for a good surgeon. In surgery, neatness counts. One of the procedures we did had a suture that seemed to exemplify the idea of neatness. We often did routine operations on pigs with hernias. You'd be amazed at how often pigs get hernias. It contradicts their image of, well, pigs, who are content to lie around all day in the mud. Given their hernia rate it would be reasonable to suspect they move heavy furniture on the side. But, as it happens, hernias are a congenital problem for porkers. Once a pig has a hernia, it's useless to a farmer for breeding purposes and too expensive to cure so OSU bought afflicted pigs from neighboring farms and we operated on them. Most of the pigs lived and were subsequently sold back to the farmers. But when they returned to the barnyard, they bore our emblem: the "vest-over-pants" suture technique. A vest-over-pants suture looks like just its name and it's used in a situation where you need a suture that's particularly strong. With this suture, the skin isn't just joined, it's overlapped so that it resists tension well. I liked the vest-over-pants suture, not just for the aptness of its name but because it was enormously satisfying to execute properly.

There was one instance where my drive for perfect neatness helped Lorraine and me in an entirely unexpected way.

About midway through our surgery course we began to work on bones. As far as I was concerned, the most important thing I learned about orthopedic work is that I hated it. Until we began our bone work, I thought I wanted to specialize in surgery. I loved "soft-tissue" work and both Lorraine and I were good at it and were getting good grades. Then came bones. I began to think of orthopedics as "boy's work." It's one aspect of veterinary medicine that really does seem to have more of a sexist bias than other areas of the profession. That's because many of the tools and techniques of bone work come from basic carpentry. The chucks, pins and lag screws were familiar to most of the men in the class because they'd worked with them before or at least had discussed them in the locker room or while tinkering with their carburetors or whatever else they were doing with their adolescences. But for most of the women, bone work was foreign territory.

It wasn't only the terminology, tools and techniques that were difficult in orthopedics. It was the stamina required for those long, tedious operations. Sometimes an orthopedic surgery took five or six hours. When working with soft tissue, the work is subtle and delicate and you have to train yourself to move with great care; everything you're handling is fragile. When you work with bones, the emphasis is quite different. Of course the work demands precision but you can't achieve your ends with delicate movements of your fingertips. You're sawing and grinding and hammering and it takes physical strength and endurance. But I didn't know all that until weeks later.

Our first orthopedic work involved pinning two fragments of a bone together. We had the bones in advance of the class and because I lived closer to the campus I took them home with me. But once I got them home I realized it would make for a much neater operation if the bones were completely clean. What, I wondered, was the best method for cleaning bones? I certainly didn't want to sandpaper them. Then I remembered my mother cooking soup. The bones that came out of that pot were as clean as could be. In fact, now that I thought of it, a few hours of boiling would no doubt produce perfect orthopedic specimens. So I got out the biggest pot I could find, filled it with water and tossed in the bones. About an hour should do the trick. I watched the first tiny bubbles break the surface and waited until there was a fine simmer going. Then, leaving the bones bubbling merrily away on the stove, I retired to my room to catch up on some chores.

I folded some laundry and organized my mountain of notebooks, enjoying the sun streaming in through the windows of my room. Then I heard the front door slam and realized Skid must be home from work. What terrific meal would she be putting together tonight, I wondered? But my dinner musings were cut short by a blood-curdling scream that sent me running from my room. It took but a few seconds to determine the cause.

Skid, after a hard day working at the OSU food service, had arrived home with a friend. They had no doubt strolled into the kitchen for a snack or perhaps because that's the first room all home-ec majors enter first, just to touch base. I could readily imagine the scene. The friend, smelling the hearty aroma that filled the house might have exclaimed, "Oh ... soup! That smells great." But Skid, who must have quickly realized that Shelley wasn't home, wasn't so easily taken in. Sally ... a pot ... cooking ... what could it mean? She sniffed the suspicious pot. In what must have seemed to her friend a strange if not pathological reaction she shrieked, "Dog bones! Dog bones! I bet they're *dog* bones."

That's my cue, I thought as I raced to the kitchen, wondering how I'd explain this situation. Maybe I could toss in some carrots and parsley and claim that Skid was being ridiculous. Maybe I could say I had no idea where the pot and the bones came from. But when I saw the horror on their faces I realized honesty was the only policy. I confirmed Skid's suspicions as her friend made herself busy examining our dinnerware pattern, too embarrassed to know which side she should be on in this contretemps. Finally I convinced Skid that by the time I was finished scouring her pot, no residue of dog bone would be detected by even the most fastidious of cooks.

The humiliation I suffered at home was forgotten the next week when I produced the bones in surgery lab. They were the cleanest, best-looking bones in class. Everyone commented on them and I felt great pride as people came over to our table to examine them. Even Lorraine was impressed, especially when I told her the secret was Skid's pot.

Our surgery class included the captain of the football team at OSU. You're allowed to play on the team for four years and, as he graduated after three years, he still had a year of glory ahead of him. Now at Ohio State, football is to many as important as life itself. Many of the professors treated him like a young god and I can't deny that sometimes their approach irritated the others. This particular football player had not only the advantage of his position but also that of size. He was a giant guy—a real hunk of valuable livestock. And he took to bone work like a hound. His soft-tissue work was fast but often messy, but on bones the class had no equal.

In this orthopedic lab we had to pin two bone fragments together. We had to grind in a pin by using a chuck. A chuck is a sort of handle that you use to twist the pin into the bone. There are more sophisticated ways to do these things—electric drills exist—but they're expensive and we were learning to do everything the hard way. I suppose that was in case we found ourselves one day without the tools and also because it helped us to understand at close range exactly which techniques worked best.

Everyone stood at their tables with their bones and after a few words from the professor we began to grind. Lorraine's head hadn't been lowered to the job more than three minutes before she whispered to me. I bent way down so I could hear her. "Sally, look at this." I looked at the pin and saw that it was already clean through the bone. We looked at one another in astonishment. Surreptitiously we scanned the room. Everyone else, including the captain of the football team, was still hard at work, grinding away in intense concentration. We bent to our bones again and I fingered the hole Lorraine had made. We came to the same conclusion at the same time. Of course! Boiling the bones had not only cleaned them but had softened them too. Instead of having to laboriously grind through the density of the bones, we found we could insert our pin into the marrow of the bone with the ease of putting a nail through a bar of soap. We'd discovered a new technique in veterinary medicine. We stifled our laughter. Within a matter of minutes we had our bones pinned, neat as could be. This was going to be an "A" bone lab. Who could blame us for strolling up to the struggling captain and asking if we could give him a hand? His expression when he saw our perfect bones, perfectly pinned, was worth every minute spent scouring Skid's pot.

Despite the thrill of that single success, it was orthopedics that kept me from becoming a surgeon. Bone work is really difficult—physically difficult—and I knew I would never make a real success of it. And as surgeons do orthopedic as well as soft tissue work, I realized that my initial ambitions of being a surgeon weren't realistic.

After the ease of the boiled bones we had our comeuppance in an orthopedic lab where we were required to wire together the jaw of a dog. These dogs were ones who had died and whose bodies had been donated to OSU vet school. Lorraine and I were, as always, determined to do a perfect job. So before our dog's jaw was broken, we chiseled a fine line down his jawbone. We figured that when the chisel was placed in the line and hit with the hammer, we'd have a clean break and a neat wiring job. But when the man with the chisel and hammer came to us he either slipped or decided to thwart us because the chisel went wide of its mark and we found ourselves with a jaw smashed to smithereens. By some miracle of physics, we seemed to have enough pieces to make up a jaw and a half.

To fix a broken jaw you must join all the pieces using wire. You drill holes in adjoining pieces and work the wire through the holes. If you have two or three pieces of bone, it's a time-consuming task. But if you have a pile of shards, you find yourself facing a challenge. Lorraine and I were dismayed but not defeated. We spent hours drilling increasingly tiny holes in increasingly tiny pieces of bone.

The rest of the class took no small satisfaction in our dilemma. They still hadn't forgiven us our boiled bones. As they finished their jaws, some of them wandered over to our table to savor our hopeless efforts. At one point Lorraine and I turned around, probably to get more wire—we used about enough to fence ten acres of pasture—and when we turned back, there had been a slight amendment made to our dog. We didn't notice it until Lorraine went to move the tongue to get better access to yet another bone shard. She gave a little tug and the tongue came out in her hand. We both gasped. Dazed from our intense concentration, it took us a few minutes to notice that there was yet another tongue in the dog's mouth. Could it be that we really were working on a two-headed monster? Were we going to have to take half of our jaw apart and begin again and try to get two jaws out of this mess? The laughter behind us told the story. But we were beyond humor.

Finally, after everyone else in the class had been long gone, we came up with our version of a mended jaw. It was together all right but it looked more like a Picasso sculpture than an anatomically correct dog jaw. The instructor examined it in silence. Then he lifted it and shook it lightly to check its stability. For a second it managed a certain stiffness and Lorraine and I breathed a sigh of relief. But then, on the gentle return swing, the jaw seemed to become fluid so that it swung in a graceful arc, hesitated for a moment and then continued swinging. Kindly, the instructor placed it on the table, no doubt fearing its total collapse. Lorraine and I smiled ruefully, hoping for a sympathy vote. But none was forthcoming. We got a "D."

"BRUCIE"

Despite the fact that I prided myself on my precision, there were times when a major miscalculation would spoil my day. For example, there was the day Lorraine and I operated on "Brucie."

We were scheduled to do one of our first large-animal surgeries. The procedure would be a gastropexy on a sheep. This is an operation where you suture the side of an animal's stomach to the abdominal wall so that the stomach won't turn over. Certain large animals, including some dogs, have a tendency to stomach torsion, a medical emergency where the stomach rotates, cutting off circulation and digestion. A gastropexy is an operation that prevents torsion.

We all trooped outside to choose one particular sheep out of a flock of about fifteen waiting unconcernedly in a large stall. Lorraine and I finally settled on a large sheep with a benign expression and a nice set of curled horns. We took our ram and brought him into the operating room to prep him, but by the time we got there all the tables were taken so we had to use a sort of pen on the floor. This arrangement might have been more comfortable for the sheep but not for us: we had to do a bit of contorting to reach our ram's appropriate parts.

One of the big debates in the animal world is over sheep versus chickens: which is dumber. I myself have never gotten involved in the analysis as I hate to take sides on emotional issues. Nonetheless, had I been able to take a picture of those sheep being operated on, they would have won the dumbness contest hands down. For this procedure the sheep are given a nerve block so that they're able to stand and be alert but are unable to feel what's happening in their interiors. The sheep that are on the operating tables—all but ours in this case—are tied into harnesses so they're standing on tables looking about as simple-mindedly as a multicelled creature can. Then, while they're standing there, chewing their cuds and trying to stay awake, you're rummaging around in their vital organs.

Lorraine and I had our ram strapped into his pen and we were sailing into the operation when the professor came by to check our work. Our patient chose that moment to work on his cha-cha and before we knew it his intestines were falling out and banging into the bars of his pen. Lorraine tried to convince him to hold still while I desperately tried to stuff organs back into his belly. Our professor, meanwhile, was observing all this with a twinkle in his eye.

"We have real field conditions here, ladies," he said. "This is what large-animal surgery is all about."

Lorraine and I exchanged looks of despair. If only the professor would amble along and check someone else's work, maybe we'd be able to recover our dignity. But, to our consternation, he lingered to watch. We'd just about gotten our ram's intestines back where they belonged when we noticed that the professor was reaching into our incision. We assumed he was checking the accuracy of our cut. Well, at least we could feel confident about that. We'd done our usual precise job. After a few minutes—minutes that seemed like hours—he looked up at us with a big smile, his hand still inside our ram. We could feel the eyes of the class upon us.

"Just palpating your ram's ovaries, ladies," he finally said.
Our ram's *ovaries*...? The rest of the class roared with
laughter. "Sheepish" is how we looked and felt when we noticed that our "ram" was missing testicles and other essential
male equipment. It turns out that horns on a sheep don't
automatically a male make. As we finished our operation on
Brucie, as we named her after our professor, I'm convinced
she added a second expression to her limited repertory: smug-
ness.

THE CAT WITH THE TASTE FOR MUSIC

It would have been clear to even the most casual observer
that veterinary students develop peculiar sensibilities about
certain things. Or perhaps it would be more accurate to say
that they start out with out-of-the ordinary attitudes and vet
school emphasizes and confirms them. For example, Skid and
Shelley could never understand how I could talk about re-
pulsive things during meals or how I could graphically describe
operations without flinching. Of course I soon censored myself
around them but their reactions made me aware of how unconscious I was of my intimate and easy relationship with life's
raw edges. If there were any students among us who still had
a vestige of squeamishness, they had to abandon it when we
took necropsy.

In the winter quarter of my junior year I began my course
in necropsy. In this course we dissected dead animals and tried
to determine the cause of their deaths. A necropsy is an important procedure in animal medicine and finally, sadly, the
last diagnostic technique available when a case was lost. Ide-
ally, a necropsy would tie up any loose ends, answer any
persistent questions. We'd send tissue samples off to the lab
for analysis and usually determine the cause of death.

We would go into the lab early in the morning and spend

hours working on the corpses of cows, horses, sheep, goats, dogs, cats and exotics. Most of them had been dead for at least twenty-four hours and had begun to decompose. Some animals like sheep would decompose very quickly because the thickness of their coats would keep their internal temperatures high. We all dreaded working with sheep. At least I was studying necropsy in the winter and had the weather on my side. I pitied the students who'd have to spend all day in that lab in the heat of the summer. In addition to the stench, which was intensified in any heat, we had to dress in a plastic apron, high rubber boots and long rubber gloves, and by the middle of each class we began to feel as if we were decomposing along with the animals.

The smell in the gray cavernous necropsy lab was revolting. In addition to the smell of the animals there was the pervasive odor of the chemical formaldehyde. We had buckets of formalin beside our tables and whenever we found an interesting tissue—one that needed to be examined more carefully—we would throw it in the bucket. The stench of the chemical would eventually begin to burn your eyes and there were times when I felt certain I would vomit.

We would go into that gloomy room with the big steel tables in our rubber clothes with our giant curved butcher-type knives and we'd have our animal on the table before us. We'd slice them open from stem to stern. We'd begin the cut under the chin and go right through the chest and belly to the anus. If we were working on a large animal, an assistant would come along and break the ribs so we could get at the organs. If we were working on the brain, or if we had a spinal case, an assistant would have to saw the skull and extract the brain so we could examine it.

I hated working on the large animals. With a small animal you felt in control because you could locate things precisely, but when you were swimming in endless loops of bowel you could completely lose your orientation and the procedure seemed overwhelming. Moreover, the large animals smelled much worse than the small. And finally, there were academic challenges to working on large animals. Large animals are hosts to seemingly hundreds of parasites. If you were doing a large animal and the professor was looking over your shoulder, you would be called on to identify any parasite you might encounter. It added tension to an already tense situation.

We did get to choose our animals and it was suggested that we work on a variety so we could get the broadest possible experience. There was a large board in the class where they listed which animals you had worked on, and if you did only small animals it would negatively affect your grade. I did put in my time on horses and cows, but whenever I could I opted for a snake or a bird or a rabbit, with apologies to Watson. Fortunately the local zoo sent us all their dead animals so that increased our selection considerably. In addition to preferring the small animals as subjects, I also thought it would be more useful for me to work on the animals I would be likely to encounter in practice.

In one particularly memorable necropsy class four of us were working on a horse. It happened to be a busy day in the lab. Across the room another group of students was working on a cow. It was one of those freak winter days that was unusually balmy—an unexpected and welcome break in the long gray winter—welcome, that is, unless you had a necropsy class that day and were yearning for sub-zero temperatures. Our horse had been dead for at least a day, perhaps more, and he was swollen with gasses. He was going to be a real challenge. Because he'd been dead for a while, his tissues had started to decompose. Instead of removing clean samples that would be easy to diagnose, we knew we would be getting mushy material and it would be very difficult to come to any conclusions.

One of our party made the first incision and opened the horse. The smell was terrible—impossible to describe. Another student accidentally punctured a loop of bowel.

Suddenly, with a whooshing sound, a geyser of fecal matter

soared into the air. Because of the high ceilings in the room, it traveled in a tall, graceful arc. Hearing the noise, everyone in the room looked up. In a split second the class knew what had happened but no one could move fast enough to save himself. A girl who was working on the cow across the room and who fortunately wore glasses, was the ultimate target. The geyser landed square in her face, covering her glasses and most of the rest of her. As one of the cattier students later said, it could have been worse but it had been the one time she had her mouth closed.

With events like that punctuating a day, you can imagine how one would gradually develop a peculiar attitude toward gross physical functions and qualities. I think that all people in the medical profession share a view of the physical that is necessarily detached. I knew that particular incident wouldn't bear repeating at home, and though the story spread through the vet school, with Dave doing a lot of the spreading, Skid and Shelley remained in blissful ignorance of how I'd spent my day.

In some ways the worst part of the necropsy class was the clean up afterward because then you weren't focusing with an academic detachment on the work at hand. First we would hose down the big slate tables, washing all the bits of tissue off and sluicing it into the drains in the floor. Then we'd scrub the stainless-steel tables and our instruments scrupulously. Any blood or tissue that remained would be bait for cockroaches and we'd have to fight an army of them in the next lab if we weren't careful. After the hosing we put useless animal parts into a giant garbage can that would slide on a track into the huge walk-in cooler that adjoined the lab. After we'd cleaned the lab and stored or disposed of our work, we'd hose down our boots and our rubber aprons, but no amount of scrubbing would entirely vanquish the smell of the formalin.

But necropsy wasn't all grotesque. Sometimes it was bizarrely funny.

One day Lorraine and I were doing a necropsy on a cat. In

so many instances we'd be frustrated because we couldn't determine the cause of death. Many cases stymied us completely. Often the animal had been dead for too long and had decomposed too much. The interesting or suspicious tissues that we had thrown in our buckets of formalin would be sent down to histopathology for further examination in the hope that that examination would yield a clue. On some cases there was nothing we could find. This is perhaps one of the most frustrating aspects of any kind of medical work. But from the minute we opened our cat, all the usual ambiguities dissolved. She was a textbook case. She was killed by a foreign body.

Foreign bodies are the big surprises of veterinary work. I've seen animals with incredible objects inside them. The previous year I'd seen an X ray of a pit bull puppy which revealed an eight-inch butcher knife in his stomach and esophagus. To this day I can't figure out how he managed to swallow it. This is not an uncommon event during the holidays when someone puts a carving knife down and in the midst of revelry doesn't notice that their dog or cat found the scent of turkey or ham irresistible. Once in school I operated on another dog to see if I could find the reason for his failing digestion. I did: four baby pacifiers lodged in his stomach.

The cat Lorraine and I were working on had fallen victim to that most insidious of cat seducers: a string. But this cat hadn't settled for just *any* string. She'd eaten what seemed to be an entire ninety-minute cassette tape, minus the plastic case.

When a cat eats a string it can be more dangerous than you might think. If the string gets caught at any point in the cat's digestive system, or even around the cat's tongue, the peristaltic action of the intestines continues to contract around the unmoving string and the intestines begin to bunch up around it like fabric gathers. Eventually the string will cut through the intestines and an infection will develop in the abdominal cavity.

Once I had a client bring in a cat who'd spent the weekend

alone getting into trouble. When the client had left his apartment, there was a helium balloon drifting on the ceiling, but in the course of time the helium had leaked out and the balloon gradually drifted to the floor. Its descent must have been tantalizing to the cat. He eventually caught the string and swallowed it. And swallowed and swallowed until the half-deflated balloon was just a swallow from his nose. When he was brought in to me he had about three inches of string tied to a balloon hanging out of his mouth. We operated on the cat and he recovered beautifully, no doubt because the string hadn't been there for long. Usually, the longer a string's in place, the worse the case. To some degree, among veterinary surgeons, "string foreign bodies" are controversial. Most will operate but I've read about surgeons who give the affected animal Laxatone, an oily substance which is ordinarily given for hair balls which is supposed to help the pet expel the foreign body.

There were no subtleties or controversies about our necropsy cat. She had eaten an unquestioned mouthful. As we cut down her abdomen, we found a giant wad of cassette tape in her stomach. We began placing bets on how far the tape would go. We followed it through her small instestine, through the valve between the small and large intestine, through the large intestine and finally to within about an inch of her anus. The tape had cut through her intestine in six or seven places. The partially digested material in the intestines had leaked into her abdominal cavity and caused an overwhelming infection. That's what had killed her.

After we had finished a necropsy on an animal, we presented our findings to the other students. We made our presentations in a sort of miniature amphitheater that had four tiers of steps which the observers would stand on. The steps faced a small pit where the presenter would stand. A rack would be wheeled into the room, like the sort of wheeled stand you might see in a bakery. It had slots for about half a dozen "cookie trays" and on those trays would be the neatly arranged results of our necropsy. We had tissue samples including slices

of lung, liver, intestine, etc., on a tray covered with a white
cloth. We would describe them and then we'd draw our conclusions about the reasons for the animal's death. Anyone was
welcome to attend these presentations. Eager freshmen were
often there and I always enjoyed seeing them because they
reminded me of how awed I'd felt when I'd been an observer
only two years before. It was one of the few occasions when
I had a tangible sense of my own progress.

We were graded on our necropsy presentations as well as
our work on the animal and there was always a palpable air
of tension and competition in the small amphitheater. When
at last it came time for our cat presentation, Lorraine did the
honors. She held the tray, lifted the cloth and began to describe
the lung, liver and heart tissues. Finally she came to the intestines. Instead of pointing to the organ sample, she lifted
the endless string of cassette tape. There was a stir in the
room. "Ladies and gentlemen," she pronounced with great
solemnity, "what we have here is a cat with a taste for music."
Lorraine paused. The audience looked thoroughly bewildered.
Freshmen turned to professors to get a clue on how to react
to this unexpected performance. What was she talking about?
Gradually smiles of enlightenment spread on the faces ranged
on the stone steps. I heard someone whisper "foreign body."
Lorraine continued. "Unfortunately it was kitty's swan song."

ROOMMATES GREAT AND SMALL

I had always thought I had the qualifications of a desirable
roommate. I'm usually genial. I'm not a great cook, but I'm
appreciative when someone else goes to the trouble. I'm not
grotesquely messy. I'm tolerant of the foibles of others and
I'm always ready for a party, your place or mine. Who could
ask for more? Indeed, Skid, Shelley and I got along famously
most of the time. But there was one thing that never failed to
cause a certain amount of friction—animals.

Skid and Shelley didn't dislike animals but they didn't really like them either. We had already agreed to live together when it became clear that Watson the rabbit was part of the deal. They endured Watson's love for houseplants but they never quite reconciled themselves to the occasional rabbit turd in the odd corner. But it was in the spring of junior year that I really tested Skid and Shelley's endurance.

As the cold, gray days of winter gave way to springtime, the new quarter of classes commenced. It was a good season for me. As the weather improved, Dave and I went on bike trips through the nearby countryside. We even took an occasional illegal dip in a local reservoir, fortunately swimming faster than the police every time. Even my classes seemed particularly good. I was especially looking forward to my first class in exotics.

In animal medicine "exotics" refers mostly to birds, lab animals and reptiles. After a couple of years of mud wrestling in rubber coveralls with cows and pigs, I imagined working with birds and reptiles would be as precise and clean as watch repair.

Most of the time in our exotics elective was spent on birds. But right before the spring break we had a speaker who brought with him some snakes from the Columbus Zoo. The idea was for us to learn snake anatomy and to give us some experience in handling snakes. Now you might wonder why the zoo would risk their valuable snakes on a class full of green students. Someone had thought of that and they'd sent snakes that were sick. Indeed the snakes were so sick they were on their last legs, so to speak. They had infectious stomatitis, more commonly known as mouth rot. Because the condition was so advanced, their prognoses were "guarded" to "poor" and I suppose the powers that be at the zoo figured with death their certain destiny, they'd be reasonably safe with us.

At the end of the lecture it was announced that the snakes would be available to anyone who wanted to take one home and try and save its life. What an opportunity! A few weeks, maybe with luck, months, to practice holding, feeding, injecting and generally caring for a snake. The odds were not good that it would survive but, still, it would be an excellent chance to get practical experience. And maybe with luck and meticulous care, it *would* survive. How could I pass this up? But on second thought, I realized that a snake could be the last straw as far as Skid and Shelley were concerned. They had survived the boiling bones, pellet-dropping rabbits and countless other transgressions. But a ten-foot boa constrictor—the snake I had my eye on—might be pushing them too far.

In fact before the exotics lecture, I had heard that some birds might be given away and I'd asked Shelley and Skid if it would be all right if I brought one home. Their answer was a swift, unanimous "No." Skid explained in detail: "I don't want something tweeting at 5 A.M. and tossing seed all over the rugs and flying around and leaving spots." Shelley was just as emphatic: "And don't tell us that you won't let it out of the cage because that's what you said about that rabbit who left little packages all over the place and ate my plants to boot. At least you can pick up rabbit packages."

There was an additional problem. I was leaving for vacation in a week and I'd be gone for a few days. Even if I could get the snake into the house I certainly couldn't convince Skid or Shelley to swab out the mouth of a boa constrictor a few times a day. Then, as I watched one of the other students claim his snake, I knew I had a solution to both problems.

Max was one of the more handsome vet students. He was tall with dark hair and had a huge smile complete with dimples. Better than that, he had a snake in his hands. Max would be my bribe to my roommates. I stopped him as he left the lecture hall, snake carrier in tow, and flashed what I hoped was a charming smile. After admiring his boa and its advanced case of infectious stomatitis, I explained to him that I really wanted to take a snake, too, but that I'd be gone for a few days at the beginning of spring break. I couldn't ask my roommates to be responsible for a sick boa. Could he possibly stop by my apartment and care for it while I was gone? It would only be a few days. Max was willing. Now all I had to do was introduce Max and the boa in just the right way to Shelley and Skid.

When Max and I arrived at my place, I asked him to leave his snake in its bag on the stoop. I figured one snake in the apartment would be enough unless I had another Max to offer at the same time. Sure enough, when Skid and Shelley saw me carrying a green garbage bag, they were immediately on guard. "Forget it, Sally" is how Skid put it. "*Whatever* it is, forget it." "But it doesn't make any noise and here's someone I'd like you to meet." It was enormously helpful to be able to turn to Max right behind me and introduce him. Suddenly, Skid and Shelley became noticeably more compliant.

Once I had their attention on Max, I made it clear that he was part of the package. The animal in the bag would stay only if they agreed, and, if they did agree, Max would come by every day while I was gone to take care of it. I could see disgust warring with lust on their faces as they looked from Max to the bag in my arms and in a few seconds it was clear things were going my way. As they scurried to get Max a beer and generally charm him, I carried the snake off to my room. By the time they thought to ask exactly what was in the bag, it was too late.

When my poor roommates finally saw the snake they were horrified. Only the thought of Max—who was already being called "the snake charmer"—saved my boa from a quiet end at the zoo. He *was* a terrible sight. Mouth rot looks like what you'd imagine and the poor fellow had a face that was peeling and foaming. The fact that his face was attached to ten feet of scaly snake didn't help his case any. I suppose the only good thing about him, in my roommates' eyes at least, was that he was too sick to move much and obviously wouldn't last long.

I had a week to work with "Stephanurus Dentatus," as I'd named him (after a giant worm that infects kidneys) before I went away. Three times a day I had to flush his mouth with peroxide. This involved wedging a tongue depressor sideways into his mouth and turning it to open his jaws. Then, with his mouth propped open, I'd swab away with peroxide on a gauze pad until his tongue and mouth were as clean as I could get them. Every third day I had to give him an injection of an antibiotic. But it turned out that the most difficult job was getting him to eat.

If Stephanurus wouldn't eat, I'd have to tube-feed him as a last resort. Hopeless as he seemed, I thought he just might have a chance to live so I was looking for every sign of recovery. Tube-feeding would have been a kind of defeat so I wanted him to eat naturally. What's natural for a snake to eat, at least a snake in captivity, is a stunned mouse. Every two or three weeks, the snake will gobble down a mouse and that's it for food for a fortnight. In fact when I told my long-suffering roommates that he wouldn't make messes or smell, I was being scrupulously honest. Because a snake eats so infrequently, he only has a bowel movement every few weeks. And it appears as a neat bundle of tiny bones and whiskers.

Now in order to feed Stephanurus I had to get a stunned mouse. So I went to a pet shop in town and asked for one. The man behind the counter reached into a crowded cage and pulled out a little white mouse by the tail. He was about to drop it into one of those white boxes favored by Chinese restaurants and pet shops when I asked him how you stun it. He gave me a quick unbelieving glance and, still holding the mouse by his tail, without a word, he swung it against the counter. Sure enough, it was a stunned mouse.

With my take-out meal by my side, I drove home as quickly as I could. The last thing I wanted was an unstunned mouse and I didn't know how long a counter to the cranium would last. I apologized to the mouse as I made my way through the streets of Columbus. It was for a good cause. When I got home I opened the box and the mouse was still flaccid. Relieved, I brought it in to the snake. Stephanurus was looking equally lackluster. "What you need, Stephanurus," I told him, "is a stunned mouse. And you're in luck." With that, I lifted the little meal by his tail and gently dropped him into Stephanurus's orange crate. This is just the sort of thing, I thought, that I couldn't have done a few years ago. It seemed an odd kind of progress to be making.

It is true that as a vet student you should discard any sentimentality you might have about animals. It simply gets in the way and slows down decisions and ultimately makes you less effective in your work. That's not to say that you must become callous; there would be no point in working to save animals' lives and keep them healthy if you were cynical about your efforts. But you must be ruthless about squeamishness or you can't function. The funny thing is that no matter how squeamish you might be when you begin vet school, you find that you toughen up almost automatically. That's because you're usually concentrating so hard on learning, remembering and noticing things that you're focusing on the tree instead of the forest. You always have a goal and that's what's on your mind. Before you know it, you're working methodically on a cow carcass in necropsy and the day arrives when you think nothing of stunning a mouse. I was certainly on my way.

If a snake is healthy, he'll grab a mouse and eat it instantly. But poor Stephanurus, sick as he was, had no appetite at all. I prodded him a bit but all he did was stare blankly ahead with his tiny snake eyes. Meanwhile, our stunned mouse was stirring and I was facing a tricky situation. If you feed a snake a live mouse, or if the mouse becomes unstunned, it's likely that it will attack the snake and bite it if it can. If that happened to Stephanurus, given his advanced state of disease and weakness, the resulting infection could overwhelm and kill him. So as the mouse began to twitch, so did I. Within a few seconds the mouse was on his little feet and I knew that I was going to have to re-stun him and fast.

All I had at hand in my room in the few seconds I had to act was a tennis racket. I'm glad no one could see me as I hopped around the orange crate, trying to stun the mouse while avoiding the snake. What Stephanurus thought of this novel method of food presentation, we'll never know. Finally, after a few ineffectual swings that only terrified the mouse, I tried a clean backhand that turned out to be the ultimate stun.

Now I had an unfed snake and a dead mouse. At least I didn't have to worry about Stephanurus being bitten by his dinner. I left the two of them alone for a few minutes but still nothing happened. Then I remembered that if a snake is sick, he often won't eat unless he's warm enough—around eighty-five degrees—because his digestive juices won't flow. So I set up a heat lamp and waited awhile to no avail. It seemed that Stephanurus was really still too sick to eat. I was disappointed but not yet defeated. I sat on my haunches watching Stephanurus and running a finger along his now-warm scaly back as I considered alternatives. Of course I could just hope for the best. But I really didn't think hoping was going to save my snake. It was going to take more than luck to get him to eat. And then I remembered. There was one last thing to do. I could make a kind of gruel and tube-feed him.

I rummaged through my mountain of textbooks until I found the one that had the correct recipe. I was filled with enthusiasm about turning a textbook recommendation into a potential life-saver for Stephanurus. I took the book into the kitchen and set it up on the counter in one of those plastic cookbook holders. Then I got Skid's blender and began to assemble the ingredients. What would Julia Child say, I thought, as I rounded up Nutrical, a caloric protein supplement, some dog food and some vitamins and tossed them into the blender. By the time I was finished I had a brown creamy soup that looked a lot like a chocolate milk shake. That chore done, I went to my room to set up what I'd need to tube-feed Stephanurus.

I heard the front door slam and later I imagined the scene as Skid and a friend entered the kitchen. The friend, new to our apartment and therefore reckless, spotted the blender and its contents and lifted the lid. She was about to sniff the mixture when Skid, knowing that I was the only one home, yelled, "NO!" so loudly that I ran pell-mell from the bedroom to see what the problem was. I arrived in the kitchen to find Skid hunched over my textbook/cookbook reading my snake-meal recipe and yelling, "*What's* in my blender?" It was amazing how Skid could divide her attention with no loss of intensity. I knew she'd gotten to the last item when she began to grab her throat and scream, "A mouse! A mouse! Oh God! A *mouse* in my blender!" The recipe had called for a mouse but even I couldn't come to grips with tossing the little creature into the blender so I'd omitted him, hoping Stephanurus wouldn't notice the subtle difference.

As you can imagine, it was tricky convincing Skid that no mouse had sullied her blender. I lifted the lid of the blender and challenged her to smell its contents. "Believe me," I said, "it smells just like dog food. Just one sniff and you'll know that no mouse is in here." She refused to examine the evidence. In fact, she was so determined that I buy her a new blender that finally I had to reach into the garbage can and pull out the little mouse. He was a sorry sight and the coffee grounds didn't make him any more presentable, but at least he won my case. Or maybe Skid just didn't want to talk about it anymore. If only a snake would eat a stunned home-ec major.

I was at last in the clear with Skid but I still had to feed Stephanurus. It's a credit to Skid that after all she endured, she was willing to help. I just couldn't hold the snake's jaws open, put the tube down his throat and at the same time squeeze mock mouse mousse from a syringe into a tube. If Skid could have found a clothespin for her nose and a blindfold for her eyes, she would have been happier but she endured squeezing the syringe until I figured Stephanurus had had enough.

I'd thought that her role in saving Stehanuris's life would have softened Skid toward him but both she and Shelley were still reluctant hosts. To be honest, I don't think they were rooting for his recovery.

Stephanurus, for his part, seemed to be improving a bit, much to my delight. One day I decided that he should be getting some exercise, so I took him out of his crate and let him explore the bathroom. The experiment went well so the next day I let him slide around the living room. Naturally, Skid and Shelley were gone at the time. Stephanurus seemed to appreciate his freedom. First he basket-wove his way around the spokes of a bicycle wheel until he'd become a living sculpture. Then he made his leisurely way around the perimeter of the rug like a gentleman out on a Sunday stroll. But when he followed the edge of the rug under the sofa I guess he decided that the dark, cave-like effect was just the ticket for a snake home and he wouldn't come out. I tried to coax him and I tried to reach for him but he'd lost interest in returning to his orange crate. Skid or Shelley could return at any minute and something had to be done.

Finally I took a deep breath and left the apartment and went next door. I knew our neighbor only to nod to but this was a perfect occasion to introduce myself. Luckily someone, a Mr. Donovan it turns out, was home. I explained to Mr. Donovan that I needed help lifting my sofa and I hated to bother him but could he come over just for a minute. Fortunately Mr. Donovan was a friendly man. He was glad to help me to do a little furniture moving. He grabbed one end of the sofa while I explained that I needed to get something out from under it. Everything was nice and neighborly until Mr. Donovan saw me hefting Stephanurus into the air. Fortunately, the snake was clear when the sofa dropped. I thought I owed Mr. Donovan an explanation so I told him about my roommates and Stephanurus. Mr. Donovan was very understanding about the whole thing and from that moment on, whenever we ran into each other, especially when Skid or Shelley were with me, he gave me a big wink.

At last it was time for my vacation. Stephanurus seemed to be doing pretty well. That and the fact that I had Max to look in on him and treat him made me feel confident about going away. Shelley and, especially, Skid were pleased to be getting another crack at Max and I figured everyone was being left in good hands.

I returned home from my vacation late at night to find Shelley and Skid chatting in the living room. Glad to see them again, I settled right in and told them all about my trip. They told me about Max's visits. He'd been there a couple of days ago to give Stephanurus his injection. He knew I'd be home soon so it was his last visit. It turned out that, much to my roommates' disappointment, Max was really more interested in the snake than them. But they bore it with no ill will. I think they'd decided that, given their experience, anyone who was going to be a vet was not exactly a bargain to live with.

We were about to turn in when Skid got a serious look on her face and announced that there was something they wanted to talk to me about. Uh oh, I thought, they met Mr. Donovan. No more exercise for Stephanurus. Skid continued, "When we agreed to let you have the snake here you promised that it wouldn't smell. Well it does smell. Maybe it dropped one of its semiannual packages or something. But would you please clean the cage so we can invite people over here again?"

I went in to check out Stephanurus. He looked none too good. I kicked the crate and he moved but in the same position he'd been in. It was as if a giant "S" had bounced a bit. It was a noble effort but Stephanurus was really too sick to have pulled through. I returned to the living room. "He stinks because he's dead, Skid," I said, knowing what effect that announcement would have. "He's dead!" Both Skid and Shelley were shrieking. "We've been living with a *dead snake* for three days! Oh God! Why us? A dead snake!" I admit I thought it was a little funny that they were so much more horrified by a dead snake than a live one.

That night I took him out to the garbage cans. The girls wouldn't sleep with him in the house and I didn't blame them. I was about to cover him, crate and all, with some newspapers. Then I remembered that Columbus, like most places, has garbage pickers who sift through the cans looking for any salvageable items. I didn't want someone to reach into Stephanurus's orange crate and die of a coronary outside our apartment, so I left Stephanurus in plain view. The next day I ran into Mr. Donovan. "Did Stephanurus die, Sally?" he wanted to know. I said that he had and when Mr. Donovan had extended his condolences I asked him how he'd known. "Well," he said ruefully, "I saw him in the can this morning."

JUNIOR SUMMER

SELECT SIRES

Junior year was over. In many ways, as I look back, it had been my favorite year. Lorraine, my surgery partner, had become one of my best friends. Skid and Shelley had endured my menagerie and we'd grown to be good friends. We'd thrown some of the best parties of all time and had many happy memories. The only disappointment of junior year was that my animals hadn't fared as well as I had. Watson had wandered off one day never to return and, despite regular search parties and the cooperation of the neighbors, we never found him. And Stephanurus had failed to respond to my intensive medical care.

That summer, my last as a vet student, was divided in half. The first half I spent at the Ohio State University Vet Clinic. We spent much of our time visiting large animals on area farms for routine medical calls and vaccinations. It was during that summer that the women in my class first experienced the special nature of being a woman in veterinary medicine. Our class was about 40 percent female but we were the first class with so many women. The year before us had had only about 20 percent. Many of the farmers we visited had never seen a woman vet. Some were friendly and accepting; others didn't trust us at all and we had to prove to them that we were qualified. This was an especially difficult challenge for some of us because our experience was so limited that the farmers usually knew more than we did.

126

One day we were palpating cows' ovaries at a farm. In order to do this you put on a long glove, add lubricant, stand behind the cow, lift its tail and put your hand in its rectum. By the time your arm has disappeared about to the elbow, you've reached the area where the ovaries are located. You then palpate the reproductive organs through the rectal wall to see if the cow is pregnant and how far along she is.

The farmer who owned this farm was deeply skeptical about having us girls up one arm to the shoulder in his livelihood. Everything went smoothly but none of us could forget that just the day before, when we'd been palpating ovaries in one of our labs, one of the women students had put her arm up the wrong orifice. It wasn't until the professor walked around and pointed out her error that she realized why she wasn't finding any ovaries.

It was also during the first half of that summer that we got even more directly involved in cow reproduction than palpating ovaries. We had done some work on bovine reproduction in school. We'd learned how to use an electric probe in the rectum of a bull to get him to ejaculate. We performed the sperm counts on the semen samples. The probe itself is quite large and on the first day of reproductive lab one of the female students had picked it up and asked what it was for. "It vibrates," said the professor. "Oh," said the student in a small voice as her face turned red as an Ohio sunset.

While studying bovine reproduction we also learned about "heat markers"—small plastic tubes of red dye that are placed just above the tail on the backs of cows. They have an adhesive backing and they stick like refrigerator magnets to the cows until they perform their function, which is to show when a cow is in heat. When the cow comes into heat she will be mounted by a bull and the mounting will break the heat marker. The red dye will spill down her back and the farmer will know that that particular cow is in heat.

The culmination of this reproductive work was when we visited Select Sires, a large farm where they keep bulls for breeding purposes. We were there mainly to observe how semen samples were taken from the bulls and, after that, we helped perform routine tests on the samples to test for venereal disease. The bulls at Select Sires were so huge they resembled flabby trucks. They were Brahma bulls, with giant humps on their backs. They even had rings in their noses. The bulls had to be carefully controlled. They were led into metal stanchions, which kept them virtually immobile. Once there, the sample was collected as someone masturbated the bull, which seemed a primitive method given the general sophistication of bovine reproduction methods.

We stood in a group, watching this intriguing demonstration, and suddenly we heard a thump. One of our group, a female student, had fainted. We revived her and treated the cut she'd gotten on her head but no one could save her from the barrage of jokes that followed. Despite her claim that she fainted from the heat, she was known forever after as the girl who swooned from excitement at Select Sires.

The second half of the summer, in North Carolina, was perhaps tamer than bovine reproduction, but no less interesting. I worked in two clinics, one in Salisbury and one in Concord, and I split my time between them.

In North Carolina I learned about certain regional calamities, including snake bites and fish hooks. My first typically regional case was a gunshot victim and it was my worst. Not because of the wound itself, but because of what it taught me about people and animals and money.

I began in North Carolina screening Saturday night emergency cases. My first emergency on my first all-night session arrived in the wee hours of Sunday morning. It had been an uneventful night of checking animals, drinking pop and paging through textbooks to brush up on what I'd do when an animal needed an emergency tracheotomy or expert catheterization. Suddenly the outside bell was ringing and the screen door slamming.

A man in a bright red hat and down vest ran in, cradling a spaniel in his arms. Blood stained his chinos and made a delicate trail across the floor as he moved toward me. He was staring at the dog as if in anger but there was deliberate tenderness in his handling of the animal. He glanced up at me only briefly, asking where he should put Hooper. I led him into the examining room, and after he settled the dog to his satisfaction on the table, he said, "He's been shot in the leg. A goddamn shame. He's my best birder."

"Well," I said as brightly as possible given the hour and the chore at hand, "Let me take a look at him."

Hooper, black and white, with the eyes that spaniels use to break hearts, lay limp on the table. Aside from his heavy panting and bloodied leg, he seemed in fine shape. I'd get an X ray. If there were no fractures, give a shot of antibiotics, clean and suture his wounds, and hang on to him for a day or two to be sure he was on the road to recovery. Then Hooper and his obviously beloved master would be back together again. With any luck, he'd be back in shape for the fall duck-hunting season.

Eager to use some of the techniques I'd been studying, I grabbed a syringe to administer an antibiotic. But Hooper's master put a heavy hand on my arm. "No need for any of that fuss, miss. Just put him right down. And can you just bill me? They have my address. I don't want to watch."

With a last loving look at Hooper, who managed to weakly wave his plumed tail, the big man in the red cap moved slowly out of the examining room. The slam of his truck door snapped me back to attention and I put Hooper into a cage for my boss to make final decisions the following morning. This was a dog that could easily have been saved.

The next day I told my boss what had happened. I explained about the hunting dog, the relatively easy case and the owner's requested outcome. What I didn't say was that I thought his patrons were a pretty wretched lot. They treated their tractors better than their beloved animals. At least they got their machinery fixed when it broke down. Hooper had been not only a good hunting dog but also a good friend.

My boss shook his head and said, almost to himself, "It must have killed him to lose Hooper...."

Sure he knew that Hooper could easily have been set to rights. My confusion must have shown on my face.

"Sally, lots of folks around here can't afford the kind of animal care you think is just routine. Sure, we could have cured Hooper but it would have cost a few hundred dollars. He knew that and he just couldn't afford it. That amount of money could be the difference between a good and a bad season for him. He's got a family to think about too. It's tough but there it is."

"Hooper," he was muttering as he went into the examining room to his first waiting appointment, "a fine birder that dog was."

Hooper was an unforgettable lesson to me, one that made me recognize how removed from actual practice the years in veterinary school can be. I was beginning to understand the sometimes cruel economics of animal care. Many people can't afford to treat their animals, even if they're beloved pets. They get routine care and often less than that. Their pets sometimes suffer for it but it's hard to find a happy solution for a poor family with a sick pet. Hooper was a first for me but I was to see countless cases like him as the years went by and I'm sure I'll continue to see them as long as I practice. At least now I'm very sensitive to the issue of money and veterinary care.

Of course affluence isn't the only regional factor that affects animal care. You find a lot more fishhooks, for example, in trout country than you do in the canyons of Manhattan. I spent probably a total of forty-eight hours that summer getting fishhooks out of paws, jowls, tails and other less likely spots. The trickiest thing about fishhook extraction is that it gets worse before it gets better. As you probably know, a fishhook is barbed at the tip. You can't simply pull it out backward or it would rip through the flesh and cause a ragged wound. The best and probably only way to get a fishhook out is to push it through the skin until the barb appears and you can cut it off. Then you can pull the unbarbed hook out the way it came in.

My most notable fishhook case involved a man, a dog and a voluminous yellow slicker. When this trio arrived in the emergency room, they looked like a circus act. It was 5 A.M. and I looked up to see various dog and human limbs peeking out of endless folds of rubberized yellow fabric. I thought the coffee and the late nights had taken their toll.

But it turned out to be a beagle, a fisherman and a raincoat joined in an uneasy marriage by a three-pronged fishhook.

Before I set to work, I glanced out the window. It was a still morning and a good thing too. If this group had tried to maneuver in a wind they would have been carried, as if by yellow spinnaker, to the borders of the state and lodged on the first tall building.

Once I'd gotten the slicker clipped into manageable pieces and was able to see what I was working on, I went to work on the hook. I worked in silence in deference to the fisherman's embarrassment. And besides, the only thing I could think about was how this had happened. First the man's forearm was liberated. Then I went to work extracting the fishhook which had completely pierced the beagle's lip. Finally the fishhook and yards of yellow slicker were stuffed into the garbage. Hours later I heard tiny wettish sounds as the rubbery stuff rearranged itself in that mysterious way of things stuffed into garbage cans. I imagined it was the laughter of hundreds of trout as they remembered the scene that sent the fisherman and the beagle to me.

HELPING HANDS

It was during my preceptorship in North Carolina that I had my first experience with an owner being on the scene during treatment. Many people ask if they can be with their pets while I do a procedure. They want to comfort the animal and I think they are also frightened of what might happen when their pet disappears behind closed doors, carried by someone in white who doesn't *really* understand the peculiarities of their best friend. I know exactly how they feel, but usually I won't allow owners to watch a procedure. Generally it's against regulations, but in fact the biggest potential problem is that sometimes when an owner catches a glimpse of blood, you've suddenly got two patients on your hands. If I ever waver from my conviction on this issue, I just remember a dramatic morning in North Carolina.

I was alone at the hospital handling emergencies. Usually there weren't many cases on Saturday morning, but on this particular day they were coming fast and furious. The first was what we refer to as a "street pizza." It was a dog, hit by a car and dragged until it looked like its nickname.

My heart always sinks when an HBC comes in. For one thing, I can't help but be irritated, if unconsciously, at the owners. In nine cases out of ten, cars aren't at fault; owners are. Dogs should be restrained and under control whenever the remote possibility of a passing car exists. There are cases of dogs that break their leashes or dogs that escape their owners in some unexpected way. Still, most people simply aren't vigilant enough at protecting their dogs from one of the biggest threats to their lives. They think their pet is happier running free or well trained enough to be trusted without restraint and that it's cruel to leash him. But that's like believing it's cruel to keep a two-year-old from doing whatever she pleases. In some instances, more common than you can imagine, the same dog can be brought in time and time again after having been hit by car after car. Owners that are irresponsible shouldn't be allowed to keep a dog.

An HBC is a real heart-stopper of an emergency. You have to assess the situation immediately and figure out what needs to be done first simply to keep the animal alive. If it was hit in the pelvis, the hip bone can break and rupture the bladder and a ruptured bladder can be life-threatening. If it was hit in the chest you can have cracked or broken ribs, or perhaps a diaphragmatic hernia, which forces the stomach or other lower organs into the chest cavity and causes potentially fatal compression of the heart and lungs. There's quite a range of HBC symptoms: bleeding in the lungs, rupturing of the spleen, broken legs, jaws and skulls, neurologic signs, shock.

That morning in North Carolina the HBC case—a young German shepherd—was in terrible shape. One look told me it would be a fight to keep it alive, and one I would most likely lose. I quickly brought the dog into the examining room and got her on the table. She was in shock, bleeding from the mouth and gasping for breath. When I took a quick look I realized that the first thing I'd have to do would be to help the dog to breathe; at that moment her air passages were too clogged with blood to pass air into her lungs.

I had done endotracheal tubing before but always as a part of a surgery when the task is neater and easier. This time I had to pass a tube into a dog's trachea which was filled with blood. Meanwhile, the dog was fast losing ground. As there was no one available to help, I took desperate measures; I went into the reception area where the owner was sitting hunched in a chair, elbows resting on his knees. I tried to size him up. He was a big man, and when he looked up at me I realized he wasn't really a man at all but a teenager. I knew he was from one of the local farms, could tell he was strong and assumed he'd be able to help me hold his dog while I struggled with the tube. He leaped up to follow me.

There was an enormous amount of blood and it was almost impossible to see where the tube was going. I made a blind stab but realized I'd missed the airway. I pulled the tube out and now it was covered with blood. The dog's pupils were dilated and nonresponsive, her gums blue, and at that moment I realized she was probably beyond saving. Even if I got her breathing in the next few seconds, she had lost so much blood, was in shock, was showing neurologic signs and no doubt had so much internal damage that it would be impossible to bring her back.

The boy's arms were now red with blood but he was holding the dog steady. As I made the second try with the tube, I heard him whisper, "Ma'am, I've never seen anything like this before." "Yeah. She's in bad shape," I responded, not really paying attention. "Really, there's a lot of blood, ma'am."

And then suddenly I saw the dog's head fall to the table and before I could realize what was happening, the boy was sinking to the floor. At the last possible second, I caught his hands in mine and we were joined across the table, one stunned vet, one dying dog and one unconscious farm boy. I suddenly grasped the import of his comments on blood.

I knew the dog was lost and I knew that I had to help the boy. But I couldn't let go or he would fall to the floor and perhaps hit his head and be in even worse shape. I yelled for help. Meanwhile, my arms were weakening—the boy weighed more than I did—and I was afraid I'd drop him so I desperately maneuvered around the table until I could grab his torso and, in small, difficult increments, lower him to the floor.

It was quite a sight that greeted the clinic aide who had just come on duty. The boy was covered with blood and slumped on the floor and I, likewise bloodied, was trying to get his head between his knees. I was forcing myself to be calm, but though I had handled dying dogs, cats with severed limbs, horses with huge lacerations and all manner of trauma to warm bodies, I'd never seen a human faint. Give a vet any gross animal emergency and they can handle it without turning a hair—but this was a human! The aide halted in the door and gasped. "Really, it's okay," I said, desperate for the aide to join me and half-convinced she'd disappear in fright. "He's just fainted." Well, it must have been the bloodiest faint in recorded history and the clinic aide was also ignorant about what to do with an unconscious human.

In the meantime the waiting room was filling with emergencies. What next? I thought. If my luck holds, the building will catch on fire. I tore into the waiting room and stood in the door, a vision in bloodied whites. "Is there a nurse or doctor here? It's an emergency." A collection of blank faces stared at me as if they didn't understand English. I suppose the whole thing was a bit of a shock. They had come here for emergency medical help and now it looked like everything was being reversed. I could see I'd have to be more explicit. "Someone's fainted. I'll help your animals but I haven't a clue what to do with a fainting human."

A woman rushed with me back to the room where the boy lay. We had no smelling salts but the woman said to try and get some sugar into him, so, with her help, we forced some grape jelly into the boy's mouth. Bubbling purple like a baby, he finally came to, sheepish and shy, and within a few minutes the hospital was back to normal, treating the creatures again.

Since that day I've seen football players, advertising executives, musicians and truck drivers faint at the sight of kitten, puppy or budgie blood. I now know that no matter how convincingly someone insists on their strong stomach—no matter how proud they are of their war experience or their stint on the ambulance shift—I can't risk taking them on as a patient and losing the original patient. So it's always "No, you'd better wait outside. It's against regulations, you know."

AMC PRECEPTORSHIP

NEW YORK, NEW YORK

It was the first day of January, a cold blustery day, and no doubt most of my fellow travelers on the flight to La Guardia were in the midst of making New Year's resolutions. I don't bother much with resolutions; I usually put my faith in on-the-spot decisions. But that afternoon I found myself resolving to make the next weeks count. I was facing the most exciting opportunity a vet student could have. I was about to begin a preceptorship at the Animal Medical Center in New York.

At the end of the fall quarter of my senior year I had made a decision that was to affect my whole career, though at the time I thought I was simply opting for an interesting way to spend part of the upcoming winter. I had applied for a preceptorship at the Animal Medical Center.

I had returned to school that fall from North Carolina eager to begin classes but, after a few weeks of routine, I was itching for a change. After all, this was my eighth year of higher education! Besides, Dave and I had broken up over the summer. He'd graduated and taken a job working at a veterinary practice in northern Ohio and it became increasingly difficult for us to be together. We also began to realize, if subconsciously, that two vets in one household could make for a terribly hectic life-style.

136

By then many of the romances and even some of the marriages in our class had broken up. Naturally I was sad that Dave was no longer part of my life. He'd filled so much of my time and my thoughts that being back on campus, but without him, had been an adjustment. But there was also the larger question of how I was going to arrange my life.... In my rare quiet moments I couldn't help but wonder what the future held. I was still determined to marry and have a family. In my dreams I could see myself returning from a shift at my own practice, greeting my husband and two children and sitting in the backyard of our country house with them as we shared tales of our various days. Dave and I had discussed marriage; I'd been the one to want to wait until after school. People change so much in the years they're in school I didn't want to make that kind of decision until I felt very sure of myself. Now the fact that things hadn't worked out with Dave didn't mean I'd never achieve my dream but it did make me feel vulnerable to the future.

I was well aware of the AMC and its reputation, as was any vet student in the United States. Many of our textbooks were written by people who worked there. And many of our professors had spent time there. Some of the AMC staff were virtual legends among OSU students. But I'd only recently learned about their preceptorship program. Some schools, like Pennsylvania, had formal relationships with the AMC and every year they would send a half dozen or so students to work as preceptors. But Ohio State had no such affiliation and so it was only by accident that I learned about the opportunity. My friend Lesley, who had worked on Plum Island and who had taken me on my first visit to the AMC the summer after my sophomore year, was applying and encouraged me to try too.

During our senior year we had what was known as an "off quarter" during which we took fifteen hours of elective courses. Students would choose electives depending on their specialties; some would take all small-animal electives, others would opt for large-animal courses. It was during this quarter that Lesley and I hoped to go to the AMC. We filled out the forms, arranged to pay our tuition through OSU and waited for word. Late in the autumn we heard we'd both been accepted. And that's how I found myself on a plane circling La Guardia airport on the first day of 1980.

Lesley and I had arranged to share an apartment with two friends who were interns at the center. I arrived at the address by cab, paid the driver and grabbed my bags out of the trunk. But when I turned to examine the building—my new home—my heart sank. I had imagined I would be living in a typical New York apartment. But my image of how New Yorkers lived came from TV shows like "The Odd Couple," and "Rhoda," gleaned in the days when I'd had time to watch television. Where was the doorman, the lobby, the awning? Instead here I was in front of a building on Sixty-first Street between First and Second avenues that would have been more familiar to "The Honeymooners" than to "The Odd Couple." It was dingy and narrow with just the barest hint of a lobby visible through the dusty windows. But the cab was gone and it was getting dark and I had no place else to go.

It was at that moment that every story of New York City crime I'd ever heard in my life came into my mind. When my seat mates on the plane learned that I was moving to New York from Ohio, they took it upon themselves to warn me not to go to Central Park, not to walk near a building on a dark street but to stick to the curb so no one hiding in a doorway could jump out and grab me, and not to list my first name in the phone book—just an initial so murderers and rapists wouldn't be tipped off that a woman lived at my address. And now here I was in "crime city" on a fast-darkening street with two suitcases and several shoulder bags that I couldn't carry at the same time and my fantasies of a doorman fast disappearing. How was I going to get the bags up to the fifth floor without an elevator, without leaving one on the street to be stolen by hordes of neighborhood thieves? This was the beginning of my life in New York, and it was an appropriate initiation to a city where nothing is easy but everything yields to ingenuity. I began a maneuver that made me feel like a mother cat moving two giant newborn kittens. I carried one bag as far as I could without letting the other out of my sight. Then I dropped the first, returned to retrieve the second and carried it as far as I could beyond the first. I repeated this ten or fifteen times until I reached my new apartment.

Despite my initial reaction, the apartment had many advantages. For one thing, it was handy to Sixty-second Street and York Avenue where the AMC is situated. As we began to work long hours, coming in early and leaving late, it was convenient to be able to spend the least possible time commuting. Another advantage was free rent. Given that the going rate for an efficiency apartment on the Upper East Side was $600 to $700 a month at that time, we counted ourselves very lucky. Our friends, two men whom Lesley and I had met at the Iowa State Convention the previous spring, were kind enough to let us stay with them for nothing but an occasional home-cooked meal, which, given our culinary abilities, was like paying us to stay with them.

But every free ride has its bumps and jolts and that apartment had its share. The first was the location of our sleeping quarters. We bunked on the floor in the kitchen. The apartment was a one-bedroom that had been coaxed into becoming a two-bedroom when one of the guys put his bed in the dining/living room. Between his room and our other host's room was a corridor doubling as a kitchen. That was our room. Neither of us had anything against sleeping in a kitchen. But New York kitchens are different from Columbus kitchens in one important aspect. If you live in a kitchen in New York, you are probably not living alone. You are most likely sharing your space with anywhere from one hundred to one million roaches. Roaches can crowd as many relatives into the back of a small spice cabinet as there are bathers on a Coney Island beach on a steamy Labor Day. Fortunately, it was winter and Lesley and I could cover our entire bodies, including our faces, for most of the night, emerging only to interrupt the roach parties for an occasional breath of air. After a few weeks we became adept at holding intense conversations while slapping at each other's sleeping bags and exposed limbs and mashing the occasional passerby into the linoleum with a sneaker heel.

An additional problem, which was a sub-problem to the roach roommates, was the fact that we were blocking the passage to the bathroom for one of our hosts. Because we were wrapped so completely at night, it was difficult for him to distinguish, as he stepped over us in the sleepy dark, what was an arm hiding from a roach and what was a sock or a fold of sleeping bag. Inevitably, he occasionally misjudged and crushed a part of one of *us* into the linoleum.

There was one final drawback to our living quarters. A cat. It's not that I dislike cats—quite the contrary—but I had never lived with a cat before and I didn't know their ways and habits. Unfortunately, this cat was not the best introduction to the charms of the feline.

That first night, after Lesley had arrived and the boys had treated us to dinner and a complete rundown on what to expect on our first day at the AMC, Lesley and I rolled out our sleeping bags. I set the alarm for an early hour and stretched out on the floor but I couldn't sleep. I was too excited. I was in New York City! And tomorrow I'd be working at the AMC! It was like living in a dream. I knew that I was fortunate to have this opportunity and I wanted my skills and knowledge to be up to snuff. As I knew I was going to be working on a cardiology service, I took my cardiology book and went into the bathroom, where I wouldn't disturb anyone, and began to study. I reread sections of the text, memorized terms I had forgotten and generally tried to brush up on anything and everything connected with the heart. I reviewed the treatment for congestive heart failure in a dog, the most common congenital heart abnormalities and reviewed EKG normals and abnormals. I was bound and determined to get off on the right foot at the AMC.

It was late when I finally made my way back to my sleeping bag and reclaimed it from the roaches. I tiptoed over Lesley and tried to slide quietly down between the covers. It was a long day, begun in another state—it seemed like another world—and it would be good finally to go to sleep. I snuggled into my sleeping bag and was about to drift off when I realized that something was amiss. My feet felt cold. In fact, they felt wet. I quietly crept out of the down tube, trying not to wake Lesley. Inching toward the wet spot, I finally got close enough to touch it. It certainly was wet. I brought my fingers to my nose. Sure enough, the sniff test yielded results. The local cat had adopted my sleeping bag as her personal litter box. So I spent the night before my debut with towels stuffed into the bottom of my sleeping bag, knees bent into a half crouch, hoping I'd be able to walk in the morning, hoping the smell would come out, hoping the cat would make her peace with me and, most of all, hoping that my preceptorship at the AMC would be a success.

DAY TO DAY AT THE AMC

My first day as a preceptor at the AMC was like hitting white water on a raft. By noontime I felt like I'd been given a shot of Adrenalin to the heart. Back at school I hadn't even been on a small-animal rotation yet, which means that, except for my summer preceptorships, I hadn't even had much clinical experience dealing with pets. But here I was with a group of fast-moving professionals who expected me to pitch in right from the beginning. I wasn't making critical decisions, but I felt like I was. I was taking histories, doing examinations and giving recommendations on treatment. And even though I was part of a team and always had someone over my shoulder with years of clinical experience, I still felt I was seeing and learning and doing more in one day at the AMC than I had in whole quarters at school.

The basic operational unit at the Animal Medical Center is the "service." A service is a group of medical personnel who work together on every case assigned them. The usual service at the AMC is made up of the head of the service, who is a staff member of the hospital, a first- and a second-year resident and usually two interns. Those people comprise the core of the service but in addition there are usually a few others, including a couple of preceptors from vet school, visiting students and visiting vets. You can also have observers who will show up for a day or two and join the crowd.

My service for my preceptorship was called Medical Service 1 or "MS1." It was a cardiology and neurology service. The day of a veterinarian at the AMC is divided into roughly two parts: rounds and clinics. First thing in the morning, the interns update our list of cases. They add any new ones that have come in during the night and been assigned to us. They check to see what blood work or X rays are pending on our current cases. By the time they've done this, everyone has gathered and we set off on rounds. We travel in a herd, moving quickly, talking all the time, tossing out ideas on treatment or diagnoses. On rounds we check on all the cases under our care. Is their medication helping? What were the results of the tests we ordered yesterday and how will they affect our course of action? Which animals will be well enough to leave the hospital today? All of this takes a few hours.

After rounds, we go to clinics. We handle animals that are brought in by appointment as well as animals that "walk in" and are assigned us. The course of clinic work depends on the time of day, season of the year, weather and phase of the moon. On a Saturday in the summer you can probably plan on being overwhelmed as people and their pets enjoy the weather. You'll get stomach torsions, heat prostrations, lacerated paw pads, animals falling out open windows and problems that have been festering all week while the owners were too busy with work to pay attention.

The main reason for the excellent depth of experience for anyone who works at the AMC is the *sheer volume* of cases that come to you in clinics. At OSU clinics we'd see just a few cases a day. Every procedure that had to be done on an animal was a big deal. People jockeyed for a chance to do things as simple as clipping nails. There was always a crowd of students around any case that was the least bit interesting. But the AMC reflected the diversity and intensity of Manhattan itself. They just kept coming. There were so many pets waiting to be treated, so many tests and procedures to do, so much to see and learn that day after day sped by in a blink of an eye. I'd look at the clock and it would be ten in the morning and the next time I looked it would be 8 P.M. After clinics we'd go back on rounds and discuss old cases as well as the new ones we'd picked up in clinics. Sometimes after one last check on the animals it would be eleven o'clock at night and I could think of nothing but falling into bed.

I remember the day I learned to do a cystocentesis. It was the second or third day of my preceptorship. We needed to get a urine sample from a female dog. A cystocentesis is a procedure where you put a needle into an animal's bladder and withdraw a urine sample. We had taken urine samples at school but we hadn't used the method preferred at the AMC. We had usually catheterized an animal to get a sample. This meant running a tube into their urethra and, for female dogs or cats in particular, it can be very uncomfortable. So now it was time for me to do a new procedure—a cystocentesis— and do it quickly.

If I had been at school learning a new procedure, we would have had a lecture on it, perhaps followed by a quiz and finally a lab where we'd get to try it. Now they just wanted the results. Someone handed me a dog and a needle. I said I didn't really feel confident about doing a cystocentesis. Someone else said she'd show me. She cradled the dog on his back, holding both rear legs in one hand. When the dog is in this position, if you drop a bit of alcohol onto her belly it will pool in a small natural indentation that happens to mark the location of the bladder. Then you just tab the needle in quickly and fill the syringe with urine so fast the animal hardly knows what has happened. I thought with chagrin of the yelps of cats and dogs as they're held in an uncomfortable position and catheterized for the same purpose. And in a few minutes I was doing a cystocentesis. I had a handful of people watching me but they weren't going to grade me, they were simply going to guide me to make sure I did it right. This was one of the most important lessons of the AMC: there was no real competition, only a demand for achievement. Everything else fell to that principle. This was really the front line.

During my years in vet school I was busy learning all about every imaginable disease of animals. The emphasis was on committing to memory the tiniest detail of a disease from pathophysiology to necropsy findings. But within my first weeks as a preceptor at the AMC I got a different perspective on animal medicine because the emphasis was on the practical or clinical approach. I saw an incredible range of ailments. I also saw what problems were the most common. As a vet you have to maintain a delicate balance between suspecting the exotic and recognizing the ordinary. You can never rule out the strange and the unexpected. Like the snake that came in because he seemed depressed and wasn't eating. Turned out he had swallowed an entire bath towel and was having difficulty digesting it. But though you're educated to a seemingly endless array of possible diseases, you have to become sophisticated about recognizing the common ones in short order so that you can save pet owners time and money.

Certain diseases we saw repeatedly—not necessarily complicated diseases but ones that seemed to be common.

Blocked cats were the first group of sick animals that I noticed were extremely common. People would come in with a male cat who was straining at the litter box, licking his genitals, producing blood in his urine or simply making frequent trips to the litter box or urinating in strange places like the bathtub. Some people would notice the problem because they would go to pick up their cat and he would scream in pain because of the tenderness of his distended bladder. As soon as we got this history, we'd be fairly certain that the cat had a urinary obstruction. Then we'd feel the belly. Usually a cat's bladder is about the size of a walnut or perhaps a bit larger if the cat hasn't been to the box in a while. But a blocked cat has a bladder that is swollen, often to the size of an orange or a grapefruit. This distension is extremely painful to the cat: thus the crying if touched.

The obstruction itself is caused by a deposit of crystals in the urethra, the thin tube that leads from the bladder. These crystals are made up primarily of magnesium and phosphorous. They form a kind of sand and, in fact, when I first heard about blocked cats during my first voluntary veterinary job after college and before vet school, the blockage was referred to as sand and I wondered if cats got it from playing in sand boxes. I often recall my confusion because so many clients think the same thing when the crystals are referred to as "sand." The crystals lodge in the urethra and they block off the flow of urine. That's why the cat will strain at the box. His bladder is large and he feels the need to urinate but is unable to.

There's some disagreement about the cause of the crystal formation. It used to be thought that the crystals became a problem in male cats who had been altered at a young age. The castration, in this view, prevented the urethra from enlarging sufficiently to let the crystals pass through. This theory has since been disproved. Some vets believe the crystals are secondary to a viral infection, but the most common and accepted theory is that urinary obstructions are related to diet. Diets that are high in what is called "ash," which really refers to mineral substance, cause the problem by encouraging the formation of the "sand." We've also come to think that any kind of stress exacerbates the problem.

We now recommend that any male cat who's had urinary problems be fed a low-ash diet. You'll notice that some cat foods will say "low ash" on the label but this can be misleading.

Cats need a certain ratio of minerals and some of the "low ash" foods are unbalanced in that they can have a very high level of magnesium. Most vets agree that canned food—not dry—is the best choice for a male with potential or past urinary problems. In fact, the AMC generally recommends either a prescription canned food called C/D, available from pet-food supply stores, or else Friskies Beef and Liver Buffet as the best choices. In addition to diet, some vets think acidifiers help decrease crystal formation. Since I've had several clients who swear that every time they take the cat off acidifiers he reblocks, I recommend them. At the AMC we recommend ammonium chloride granules: one-quarter teaspoon daily mixed with the food. Usually the cat will eat the food plus the granules without problem. We also suggest that owners lightly sprinkle the cat's food with salt. This makes the cat want to drink more, urinate more and keeps the fluids and possible sand thinned out and moving through the system.

The real tragedy of a blockage in a cat is that a cat who has been blocked for more than twenty-four hours is a critical case and sometimes a lost one because the toxins in the urine get absorbed into the bloodstream, affect the heart and can kill the animal. That's why it's important to remember, particularly if your cat has been blocked in the past, never to leave him alone for a long period of time, like a weekend, without having someone to look in on him once or twice. I've seen cats die with blockages because they've been alone for several days and there was no one to notice their symptoms.

The treatment for a blocked cat is catheterization of the bladder. Once catheterized, the urine passes and then the bladder is flushed out with a solution enabling the sand to pass.

Blockages in cats was one of the first ailments that I noticed as being especially common. But it was also one of the first that I realized could be readily avoided. Some cats came in two or three or more times with blockages, and if their owners had payed more attention to diet, they could have avoided a great deal of discomfort on the part of their cat and expense on their own behalf. Some cats may continue to reblock even though the owners feed them a low-ash diet and acidifiers. These cats are candidates for a surgery to dilate the urethra so they can pass the sand. But most can be helped with a careful diet.

In addition to blocked cats, there were other pet ailments that revealed themselves as being unfortunately frequent. One of the worst and most common even had its own nickname: "The New York Spay."

In most parts of the country, people will spay their female dogs when they're young. But, for some reason, many people in New York never bother to have their dogs spayed at all. As the dog gets older many of these intact females develop an infected uterus. Pyometra is the name of this condition and it most commonly occurs in dogs over the age of seven years, although I have seen it in younger dogs. The owner may notice that the dog won't eat but it will usually drink a lot of water and urinate frequently. Often the abdomen is distended. The symptoms most commonly begin two to three weeks after being in heat. As the infection worsens, the dog, or cat, gets sicker. They become anorexic, they begin to vomit, may have diarrhea and they become listless. Pyometra is a serious and potentially fatal condition which has to be corrected by surgery. The surgery is a spay but it's more involved than a regular spay on a healthy dog. The dog is sick and anesthetic risks are greater. There's also more chance for postoperative infection since the surgery is being done on infected organs. If brought in early enough, however, the dog usually does well. Because vets see case after case of pyometra at the AMC they came to call the surgery a "New York Spay," and we always hated to see one come in because it was a condition that could have been prevented by spaying the animal when it was young.

As the days went by at the AMC certain cases like pyometras and blocked cats became routine and I could spot one quickly and handle it readily. I was developing more proficiency than even I knew and I wouldn't really appreciate how much and how quickly I was learning until I left the AMC. A good vet is, of course, knowledgeable about a myriad of diseases and can survey a history and a set of symptoms and come up with a disease. But there's also an instinct at work and *that's* the art of veterinary medicine. It was while I was at the AMC that I realized that some vets have a gift for this but few vets can develop their gift or instinct without lots of experience. The AMC had the enormous volume of cases that provided a rich background. If you paid attention you absorbed so much information that when the time came you could draw from your experience and see the common disease with unusual symptoms or the unexpected rare disease that lurked behind a few simple clues.

In addition to the volume of cases, the AMC boasted just about the best people in the business. I remember on my third day being introduced to Dr. Tilley. I knew that Dr. Tilley was on our service but he hadn't been around. Suddenly this tall guy wearing sneakers and round glasses was introduced to me as Dr. Tilley. It took me a few minutes to realize that this was "the" Dr. Tilley, the man who had written the cardiology textbook I'd been studying so hard only a few nights before. All I could think to say was, "You don't look old enough to have written a book." He laughed with pleasure. He must have been used to awed preceptors staring at him. Here was a man who was tops in the field and he was taking his time to show me how to take and read EKG's on cats and dogs. And he was happy to answer my questions on anything. And, best of all, I got to watch him and other experts do what they did best. I became a willing sponge because I knew right away that I'd never have a better chance to absorb information than right then and right there.

One of the first things I noticed at the AMC was the atmosphere. It was intense and fast and there was a great tolerance for eccentricity. Coming from Ohio, I was unprepared for New York–style jokes and familiarities. For example there was one vet at the AMC who would rush up to pregnant women and lightly press his hand to their bellies. It didn't matter if the woman was a total stranger. As the woman stood, usually stunned, he would announce "boy," or "girl." He'd bet the mother a dollar that his analysis would be right. The peculiar thing is that he usually was. Every now and again he'd run around the clinics waving a dollar bill in his hand. Another mother would be paying up.

There was another vet who insisted on referring to all pets as "she." It was just a habit he'd developed and one he couldn't or wouldn't break. It was "She needs a castration" and "She's got a prostate infection" and that's all there was to it. I noticed that some vets just chose a sex and referred to all their patients by either he or she. I thought it was a strange practice until I found myself doing the same thing. It wasn't deliberate. It was just a matter of concentration. I was so busy concentrating on the diagnosis and treatment of the animal that I didn't concentrate on which gender I was using when speaking about the pet. The goal was always the best care and cure of the animal; anything that wasn't essential to that fell by the wayside.

CATS IN LOVE

There was a wonderful feeling of camaraderie among the staff members at the AMC. I suppose it's like being a war correspondent. So much is happening to you and it's happening so fast and no one can really understand it unless they're going through it too. You're sharing fears and experiences and, particularly if you're a preceptor, knowledge.

For example there was the night that Lesley and I were trying to sleep with a cat in heat. Our time on the kitchen floor had run out and we had to search for an alternative place to stay. Someone at the AMC told us about an intern who was going on vacation and needed someone to house-sit for him. He would be gone for two weeks. It was a perfect setup for us and so Lesley and I gathered our things and, like no-mads, prepared to pitch our tents a few blocks away. There was only one drawback to this new arrangement and I was determined to be broad-minded about it. Despite my experience with the other interns' cat, I was not going to be bothered by the one living in our new apartment. I was going to make friends with it and the three of us—Lesley, the cat and myself—were going to have a blissful two weeks together.

The first evening after work, everything seemed promising. Lesley and I had been at the AMC late that night and were both exhausted. We came home and sat in our new living room, relishing the prospect of our first night in New York to be spent in a real bed. It would be heavenly to hear springs squeak beneath us, to be high on a platform safe from serendipitous cockroaches. Even the cat seemed welcoming. She purred when we petted her and rubbed up against our legs with enthusiasm.

But it seemed kitty wasn't tired. Or perhaps she'd been lonely after a solitary day. Whatever the reason, it was clear she wanted attention. Relentlessly she paced the length of my bed. She pawed my face. She padded my stomach. And finally, frustrated with the lack of response, she began to yowl. She cried and cried. She was in misery. But she was no less miserable than Lesley and I, and we convened in the living room to discuss our roommate. It took the two of us, both vet students, a relatively short time to realize that our little friend was in heat. We knew all about cats in heat from clinical experience. We knew the hormone levels that determine heats, or "estrus" as they are technically known, depend on the hours of daylight. Cats from the southern latitudes go into heat more frequently than northern cats. We were grateful that we were not preceptors at Tahiti Medical Center.

We also knew that nature cares more about cat reproduction than human peace of mind. Cats can be in heat for about two to three weeks and they begin to exhibit signs a few days before they're ready to mate. That's a holdover from the days when cats in the wild lived far away from each other. A female in heat had to send out the signals way in advance if she wanted to find a suitable mate by the time she was ready to reproduce. The signs of estrus in a female cat are not difficult to recognize. She will rub herself against people and anything else that holds still for a few minutes. And she'll spend a lot of time with her rump in the air, treading with her rear paws and flinging her upright tail side to side. The most significant sign of heat is the "cry" of the female, whence the term caterwauling. We were being treated to full-throated caterwauling and I was beginning to think that male cats would rush to mate with a female in heat if only to shut her up.

It was an experience that threatened to sour us on our new digs, and in fact we were beginning to think that the owner of the apartment might have calculated his vacation to coincide with kitty's heat. When you begin to have such uncharitable notions it's time for a plan of action. But all Lesley and I could think to do was to put the cat in the kitchen for the night, crawl under our respective covers and bury our heads in our pillows. I was beginning to long for the peace and quiet of hordes of pillaging roaches.

The next morning we released the cat and rushed to work, leaving her to her own devices. I considered putting the television on so she could watch "The Dating Game," but Lesley vetoed this as unprofessional. So there we were at the AMC, earlier than we'd ever been and more tired too. But we weren't working in the most sophisticated, technically advanced animal medical center in the world for nothing. Before we could get even a fraction of the sympathy we felt we deserved, a resident came up with a solution: "Probe 'er." Would it work? Of course it will work, he insisted. Do it as soon as you get home.

By the time we arrived home that night we'd almost forgotten about our desperate friend. But the second we came in the door, she reminded us of her single-hood. Despite the fact that we were all in the same boat as far as that was concerned, our sympathy quickly dissolved. It was time for the resident's solution.

We brought out the equipment and went to work. First the

sterile thermometer that we had brought from work. Then
the sterile vaseline recommended by our friend. Then we took
the thermometer and proceeded to "probe 'er" by gently in-
serting the tip of the thermometer into her vagina and thrusting
it back and forth several times. By taking on the role of a male
cat, we induced ovulation. Shortly after the cat ovulates, she
ceases her heat behavior. In a matter of time, kitty was happy
and we were able to get a good night's sleep.

THE LLAMAS OF THE BRONX

About midway through my AMC preceptorship I was
scheduled to do a rotation at the Bronx Zoo. I had done some
work with zoo animals in Ohio but that had been one day at
a time and I never got the real flavor of working with the
exotics day after day.

I was eager to be at the zoo but terrified about getting there.
I'd been in New York long enough to get across town and I
knew a few subway routes, but the trip to the Bronx Zoo was
to another borough! I was explaining my cowardly feelings
one morning to two friends at the AMC and they decided that
we'd all do a dry run together the next morning—the day
before I began work at the zoo. We boarded the correct subway
and rode for what seemed to be quite a long time and then
the train, which had been hurtling along through the dark
tunnels beneath the streets of New York, was suddenly in
daylight. I thought that perhaps we'd landed on a roller-coaster
track and now would begin to do a double loop. Or maybe
this was old abandoned track and we'd soon be hurtling into
the East River. Seeing my alarm, my friends explained that
some of the subway lines turned into regular everyday above-
ground trains when they reached a certain point and this was
one. Reassured, I began to enjoy the unusual sensation of
riding a subway in broad daylight.

The next morning it was time for me to try it alone. I got up very early: I had to be at the zoo by eight o'clock so I figured that if I left by six-thirty I'd make it on time. I'd planned to use my old, beat-up stethoscope but I'd left it in my locker at the AMC, so I grabbed the shiny new one my parents had given me for my birthday, stuffed it into the pocket of my down parka and ran for the train.

Riding the rush-hour subway in Manhattan is something I'd never tried before and once I pressed my way on to the car it struck me as an appropriate beginning for a day at the zoo. The noise level was tremendous and I realized why I commonly saw New Yorkers wearing Walkmen or earplugs.

By the time we emerged into the light, the crowd had thinned out and I regained the ability to move my head at will. As we continued to hurtle along and I surveyed the crowd I began to realize with a sinking feeling that yesterday's trip to the zoo would not be the help I had expected. We had been having so much fun talking and laughing that I hadn't really noticed how long it had taken to get to the zoo and what stop we'd gotten off at. I was mulling this over and wondering what happened when the subway reached the end of the line— did it just stop and abandon you?—when we lurched to a halt at a stop marked "Bronx Zoo." I leaped from my seat and onto the platform just as the doors closed.

But two things were wrong. It wasn't the stop we'd gotten off at yesterday. And my stethoscope was gone. I remembered how pleased I'd been when my parents had given it to me. Though I'm sure that sometimes they wished I'd just settle down, forget vet school and get married, they were always supportive of my efforts, and the gift of the stethoscope had been symbolic to me. It had been brand-new, expensive and I'd never even gotten to use it. Besides, could I even tell my parents what had happened to it? One had to be very careful explaining New York's daily traumas to one's parents from Ohio. I had that terrible sense of anger and frustration that comes from being a victim. But the more immediate problem was getting to the zoo, which seemed nowhere in sight. I finally found someone to ask and she told me that I'd have to take a bus a few blocks away and ride it for ten or fifteen minutes. When I finally arrived at the giant gates of the zoo they were locked. It was the last straw. I began to cry. Surely passersby wondered why a grown woman would be so disappointed that the zoo wasn't open yet.

From that low point my week at the zoo was all uphill. I visited the Bronx llamas with special pleasure because I knew I wouldn't have to work with them. My experience with llamas at the Columbus Zoo had been unforgettable. One day during my brief stint at the Columbus Zoo we had been charged with rounding up the llamas, who were to be moved to a new habitat. This had sounded like fun. I imagined the llamas, cute and furry and ever so grateful to be getting a new spacious home. It turned out that llamas can be very contrary about moving and are oblivious to the finer points of environmental decor. They seemed to be determined to stay right where they were.

Eight of us—the zoo vet, myself, three vet students and four animal handlers—had spent the better part of a day roping llamas and I gained a new understanding of why cowboys are so eager for that first beer after a hard day on the range. Roping's hard dusty work. For us it was also dangerous. We had a spear tipped with a narcotic called M-99 which we would bring into play if one of the llamas became violent. While the M-99 would act to sedate the llama, if one of us got pricked with the spear we could die. It had happened in the past, so the rumors went, and we'd all discussed it before the big roundup. We spent a lot of time avoiding the spear.

Capturing the llamas meant lassoing them, then dragging them onto a truck. They reared and kicked, and every time we got one on the truck it was cause for celebration. Finally, after hours of work, we had gotten the whole crew aboard and dropped the back panel into place. It was a great moment in llama-moving history. But the most amusing moment was yet to come. When we drove the llamas to their new digs and lifted the panel to free them, they left the truck in an orderly line, suddenly as docile as schoolchildren entering a museum. Without a kick or a sound, they made their way into their new habitat and stood in a group looking at us with great puzzlement, as if to ask what all the fuss had been about. The Bronx llamas seemed docile and compliant, but I knew that it was all a facade.

My time at the Bronx Zoo was spent working with animals who were more cooperative. There was an anteater who had demodectic mange, and an elephant with a bruised trunk and a bear who needed a tooth pulled. A bear with a toothache is a frightening animal and we had to use a dart gun to sedate him. Like most people, I used to think that you just aim and shoot with a dart gun and the animal slumps immediately to the ground. But you have to take aim very carefully. If you hit a nerve or some other dangerous spot you can seriously damage the animal. The goal with the bear was to get the dart into the large muscle in his back. As you might imagine, he wasn't eager to turn around and hold still so we could get a good shot. But eventually he did and we aimed, shot and hoped. The dart went home and after a few seconds the bear slipped to the floor and we could go to work.

Zoo work was a memorable experience. I missed the personal contact with owners that I usually found so enjoyable. When the week at the zoo was over I left without any real regrets.

SENIOR YEAR

OSU AGAIN

The real benefits of my preceptorship became quickly apparent to me in my first days back at school. Everything seemed easier. I had a new confidence that came from experience. For the first time I was the student people would gather around as I demonstrated a tricky technique that had become second nature to me by virtue of endless repetition under sometimes trying conditions in New York.

I remembered how, at the end of junior year, which now seemed eons ago, when we'd go on rounds in the clinics the seniors had seemed to me like gods. We, as juniors, were there to observe and so we'd try to blend unobtrusively into the background and absorb as much as we could. The senior would get the animal's history from the owners and then examine it. Then he'd go into the hall and discuss his diagnosis with the staff member. I remember well the day I was with a senior who examined a dog, got a quick history and then returned to discuss the case with the staff member. "What do you think it is?" asked the clinician. "Lympho," said the senior. "Right," said the clinician. I was amazed. He'd diagnosed it as lymphosarcoma in about ten seconds flat. I had studied the disease but I wondered if, under the same circumstances, I would ever have come up with that diagnosis. I asked the senior how he did it and he told me, "Don't worry. When you're a senior, you'll be able to do it too." I hadn't believed him, but now, for the first time, I knew he had been right. At last it seemed likely that when the time came for me to face the real world, I could do it.

PIGS, BEGINNING TO END

There is a branch of veterinary medicine that inspects live-stock that is destined for human consumption. Strict govern-ment standards ensure that the meat sold to consumers is disease-free and it's the job of specially trained vets to ensure that these standards are upheld. In the spring of our senior year we went on what might be called a field trip to visit a meat-packing plant and learn more about the job of meat in-spection.

The plant we visited packed pigs. In walked hordes of squealers and out came pork rinds, sausages, hot dogs and bacon. The actual processing part was a pretty grisly sequence of events. First the pigs emerged from pens and were forced single-file up a ramp. At the top of the ramp each pig would be stunned. Then one of their hind legs would be hooked on to a chain that hung from a moving pulley and, almost as soon as their bodies were hoisted into the air, their throats would be slit so that they would bleed out from the jugular vein. So within the space of a few minutes, before we could really adjust to what was happening, we were watching a line of upside-down pigs bleeding from the throat.

As the pulleys moved across the vast room, the pigs reached a boiling-hot bath at just the time that they should have been bled out. At that point the pulley track dipped so the pigs could be submerged in scalding water. The high temperature of the water loosened their hair follicles so that their hair would come out more easily.

After their bath the pig carcasses, still hanging upside down on the pulleys, go through a sort of procedure that resembles an automatic car wash but instead of brushes there are paddles that hit the pigs and remove the hairs. It's a peculiar sight, the line of pigs swinging to a rhythm set by the smacking sound of the paddles. Finally the carcasses reach their last station, which is fire. They go through a sort of corridor of flames that singe off any remaining hairs. As their bulky shapes travel through the corridor, you can see occasional leaps of blue flame where a hair that the paddles missed is burned. Finally the carcasses emerge from all these treatments, dead, clean and hairless and very very pink.

After processing, the carcasses go through another sort of assembly line where they are cut apart. This was the most interesting part of the day to us because there was a veterinarian on duty who pointed out to us any abnormalities or diseases he discovered. For example, there's a bacterial disease of pigs that causes diamond-shaped lesions on the skin. The vet discovered a case or two. Of course, the entire animal was condemned and stamped as unusable. The healthy animals continued on the assembly line to their futures as processed food.

On the assembly line each worker was responsible for a specific part of the pig. One woman might cut off just the head; another might be amassing a pile of stomachs or spleens. If one worker turned to talk to his or her neighbor for a minute, there would be an offal pileup that then had to be dealt with double-time.

I'd heard that every part of a pig is used except the squeak and it's true. The fat, the eyes, the rind, the feet, the ears, even the pancreas, which is used for insulin—*everything* was processed into some useful form. To be honest, most of us found the tour revolting and there was much talk of vegetarianism throughout the day. In my opinion pigs are not sympathetic creatures. Still, it's terrible to watch them being turned into pork rinds. The flames, the bloodbath, the boiling water, the paddles—all of those procedures seemed so dramatically at odds with the work we'd been training to do. Our main interest was to save animals' lives.

In a curious way the worst part of the day was the moment at the very end when you emerged from the processing room to find a smorgasbord of pig products offered for your enjoyment. Hot dogs, fried pork rinds, bacon—anything deliciously piggy was there for the taking. We looked, dumbfounded, from the wieners to one another. Taking the measure of that neat pink line, I'd bet that more than half the people in the room, more than half the people who ever pass through that room, vow never again to munch on a frank.

CAMP AMERICA

Toward the end of our senior year we all faced the last two hurdles we'd have to clear before we were full-fledged veterinarians. We had to pass both the national boards and the state boards in the state where we intended to work—for most of us, the Ohio State Boards. Both sets of boards are long, complicated, difficult exams designed to test you on everything you've learned in four years of school. The Ohio State Boards had been instituted the previous year—before that there were no Ohio boards—and one third of the class had flunked. We were the second group to take the test. Most people passed the national boards but they were still a challenge. They were psychologically grueling because if you failed them you couldn't practice anywhere.

The only weapon against the formidable opponent of the combined boards was study and lots of it. My first gesture toward preparation was a failure. I decided to join a study group. Such groups were forming all over school. We had copies of previous national boards and each person would be assigned a certain number of questions to investigate. When we got together, we'd go over everyone's answers. My group consisted of four people: Lorraine, myself, one other student and the smartest person in our class, Jackie Jenkins. We congratulated ourselves on being in a study group that could boast as a member the girl who eventually graduated first in our class. We figured it couldn't help but rub off. A few weeks of hard work with our study group and we'd be in the clear.

I should mention here how we got copies of previous board exams. Of course we weren't supposed to have them but as at many colleges and universities, there was a tradition that seniors would give juniors the questions that they'd been asked on the boards. Before the test each senior was given a number that they would be responsible for. For example, if you had the number "2" you were responsible for remembering every question that ended with a "2," which would include questions number 2, 102, 302 and so on. As the seniors emerged from the test, the smiling juniors would be waiting with coffee and doughnuts. But before each senior got their refreshment, they had to report the questions they were responsible for. They didn't volunteer the answers; that wouldn't have been sporting. And of course to the faculty it looked like the juniors were once again supporting the class before them by donating doughnuts and coffee to cheer the spirits of the outgoing class. The National Board Committee has since tightened up on this practice: they change the tests every year and they began with our year. So all our coffee and doughnuts went for naught.

The first thing we learned in our study group is that studying is like playing tennis; if you want to do well, work with people at your own level. If your comrades are below you in ability, you'll become cocky and impatient. If, on the other hand, you're training with a champion, you'll quickly get discouraged. I'm afraid our predicament was the latter. We would arrive at study group, each prepared with her material. Lorraine and I and the other student would move slowly through our areas, reasoning and explaining, leading the rest of the group to our conclusions. But the brilliant member of our group was so familiar with the material she'd roll answers off the cuff and leave us gasping. In addition to being very smart, Jackie had a photographic memory. The convolutions we endured to get bits of information imbedded in our brains were foreign to her.

After a few weeks of the study group, Lorraine and I decided that we had to find a better way. As it happens both of us had the spring break off. When you're a senior you're responsible for the cases at the OSU animal clinic so you have to be there all the time. You have no vacations because students have to be there to care for the animals. But the school does have a system of rotation so that every senior gets one of the breaks—Christmas or spring break—off. As Lorraine and I both had the spring break free, we decided we'd use that time for intensive gunning.

Certainly there was no point in staying on campus when we didn't have to be there. We thought it would be ingenious to combine vacationing and studying into one grand marathon. It didn't take us long to realize we were facing an opportunity to take part in the great American collegiate dream: spring break in Florida. It would be perfect. We'd take all our materials, drive down to Florida, studying all the way of course, and then spend ten days dividing ourselves between intensive work and intensive fun. We'd return to school smart and tan and the envy of our classmates.

As you might imagine, everyone was skeptical. No one could believe we'd really get any studying done. No one could believe we'd make it to Florida in Lorraine's old van. And no one could believe that we'd get a hotel room. It was that last objection that began to worry us. What if we couldn't find a place to stay? The dream of the perfect spring break began to fade. Depressed and discouraged, we regrouped. The morning of our intended departure we hatched a new plan. If we couldn't go to Miami, Florida, we'd to to Miami University, Ohio. Miami University, site of my undergraduate education, would be a suitable alternative. And besides, if we went there, we'd never have to tell our classmates that we hadn't made it to Florida; we'd be able to say, of course we went to Miami.

Our ultimate destination was Camp America. Camp America is a state park near Hueston Woods, which is a stone's throw from Miami University. People come to Camp America and rent cabins to enjoy the fresh air, the woods and all the activities that go hand in hand with a week away from it all. Lorraine and I figured that, though it wasn't Florida by a long shot, at least it was a place where we could study. Into Lorraine's van went all the documentation of three and a half years of learning. For each class we had a three-inch stack of notes in a binder. As we usually had five or six classes per quarter and three quarters that meant we had fifteen binders per year for a grand total of sixty notebooks. Each notebook was piled into the van. Then there were the textbooks: histology, embryology, ophthalmology, anatomy and so on. None of these textbooks were lightweights. I suppose all told we had about eight feet worth of stacked textbooks. Into the van they went. Then we had to think about furniture. If we were going to stay in a small cabin, we couldn't expect to find the facilities of a study lab at a major university. So we loaded folding tables and chairs into the van on top of the notebooks and textbooks. We brought everything we could possibly need for what we anticipated would be ten of the grimmest days of our lives and we were the talk of the campus as Lorraine and I and a half ton of study supplies disappeared over the horizon.

Pulling into Camp America a few hours later, our hearts were faint. Would we really be able to study harder than we ever had in our lives? Would we really learn enough to pass both the state and the national boards? Would we really be able to fit all the stuff in the van into a cabin? The drive had dampened our enthusiasm. We stumbled into the camp office to learn which cabin we'd been assigned. "Cabins aren't open yet, ladies," said the man behind the desk. "Too early in the season." "But we called this morning...." Lorraine and I exchanged desperate glances. We really *had* called. "Yes, I remember your calling and we're going to put you in the mess-hall cabin if that'll be okay. It's five dollars per person per night and you can have the whole cabin except for Saturday night, when there's a wedding reception. You'll have to clear out for that night."

Lorraine and I found our way to the mess-hall cabin. When we opened the door, much to our surprise and delight, we found the most perfect setup imaginable. There were eight long tables where we could put our books. There were enough chairs to seat the Chinese Army. There were bunk beds and multiple showers. And, for those midnight snacks, there were cans of Campbell's soup as big as Cairn terriers. And finally, for those moments when a diversion was essential, there were pinball machines set to work at the push of a button. If we'd paid for all the pinball games we played during that study session, it would have been an expensive week. We were in study heaven. We spent the rest of that first day unloading the van and arranging the materials. We lined up the textbooks and the notebooks in order all along the length of the tables and we figured that if we moved along them at the rate of half a table per day we would have covered every possible subject in veterinary medicine within our allotted time.

The days passed just as planned. We got up early every morning and began studying. We worked like demons. No detail escaped our attention. We moved easily from ophthalmology to hematology to respiratory to cardiology to pharmacology to digestive and integument. After a few hours of work we'd break for lunch and a few passes at the pinball machines and then we'd be back at the books. Late in the afternoon we'd take a running break. Lorraine had never done much running and, sensible girl that she is, she couldn't understand running without a destination so every day we'd run to the ice-cream parlor in town, have some ice cream and run back. We became familiar figures as we panted our sweaty way to the counter each day.

After ten days of studying and running, Lorraine and I felt we'd accomplished our goal. We had taken almost every course and condensed the important information into a couple of little black books. Working eight to ten hours a day, we'd covered nearly everything we'd ever learned and some things we hadn't. The only thing we hadn't done was get a tan. It was going to be difficult to maintain the illusion that we'd spent spring break in Florida with our pale faces so for the last few days of our stay at Camp America we bought a sun lamp. Every day we'd spend some time under the lamp reciting drug dosages. By the time we packed up our half ton of books and notes, we both had a reasonable amount of color. Not really a tan but enough to testify to the fact that we'd gotten in some beach time between study sessions.

In the final analysis, the only one that counts, our ten days at Camp America were a success. The board exams, both given over a two-day period, were grueling and exasperating. Some of the questions were so technical and picayune that we could only shake our heads when we came to them. There were questions about rabbits and sharks and one about the sinuses of a horse that stumped even the class equine expert. But months later, when Camp America was a fond memory, Lorraine and I both learned that we had passed both the Ohio State and the national boards. Our unconventional "Florida" break had been a triumph.

THE BEST GIFT OF ALL

Vet school was ending. Graduation was breaking up the class that produced the Rodent and Allen. All the memories of those four years came back in the last weeks of school, and conversations were constantly sidetracked by anecdotes from the past. Once one of us had left a client with his pet in one of the examining rooms and had forgotten about them. Early in the evening, someone checking the rooms found the client asleep with his dog. We remembered the time Lorraine and I had terrified some freshmen on Halloween night. We were in the anatomy cooler and the freshmen were studying in an adjoining room. Dressed in a witch's costume, I climbed on a horse carcass which was hanging from the tracks on the ceiling. Lorraine dimmed the lights in the other room and, with several co-conspirators, swung open the doors and pushed me, yelling like a banshee, and the horse into their midst.

I remembered how our patients sometimes turned on us. There was the day in avian class when we were all handed brown paper bags, each containing a parakeet. When I gingerly reached into mine I felt a stinging bite on the finger and, in my amazement, I let out a resounding "OW!" dropped the bag and watched with the rest of the class as my bird darted and swooped through the lecture hall taking sweet revenge for his bagged brethren.

But it wasn't only the hijinks we recalled. Not one of us had escaped defeat. We had all inevitably lost surgery patients and we recalled them with sorrow and a sense of failure. Happily, there were also those patients who became our favorite cases—the abandoned animals, destined to be put to sleep for one reason or another, that we'd stolen from the school and found homes for. Of course this was forbidden— we'd risked expulsion to do it—but it was always worth the risk. Most of all we thought about the people—the professor who drew anatomical examples on female students and the one who spoke with such a strong accent that I spent the beginning of freshman year thinking I was learning about the "mudbrain" when in fact we were studying the "midbrain." The friends...so many of us had arrived four years ago as strangers. It now seemed odd that there was ever a time in my life that I hadn't known Lorraine, Lesley, Dave, Skid and Donna.

So many things had happened to me in those four years from the difficulty I'd had getting my first volunteer job to those heady days as a preceptor at the AMC. I remembered how, during my sophomore year, I was so upset because I'd left my hematology notes at school for a test the following day that even a blizzard that sent the National Guard out couldn't keep me inside. In a snowmobile suit I'd walked through miles of waist-high snow to retrieve my materials. Despite a power failure, the reflection of the moonlight off the snow made a bright and beautiful night. But the familiar landscape was disguised—no streets, no landmarks—just endless fields of snow and white-capped houses. Looking back, I could see why the police who stopped me were so incredulous about my mission. They couldn't have understood how much I wanted to study for that test, how eager I was to do well at school.

We were all feeling mellow those last days but Lorraine and I were *forced* to be nostalgic because we had been selected to put together the slide show for an evening of entertainment known as the annual "Senior Send-Off." We had only a week or so to take candid photos of everyone in the class and arrange a slide show with an amusing narration.

The day of Senior Send-Off began with Lorraine and me and a friend sitting on the floor of my apartment with a slide projector and a few hundred candids of our classmates. We arranged the slides in an artistic sequence and wrote and recorded a narration that had, in our opinion at least, all the earmarks of the best of the Hollywood roasts.

There was a feeling of eagerness verging on hysteria in the banquet hall. Finally we got the projector and the tape going in sequence and everyone settled into watching highlights of the past four years.

The slides were amusing but it was really the commentary that drew the whole thing together. For example, there was the vet student who asked out any girl who was warm to the touch and could walk. By the time we graduated, he'd pestered every single woman in the class, so his slide showed a photo of him crouched in one of the cages in the wards we used for large dogs. He had willingly crawled into the cage for the photo but what he didn't know was that we had attached a sign to the front of it. We had a batch of standard signs that we used regularly that had warnings like "Do Not Feed" or "No Liquids" or "Bites." For our Romeo we made up an official-looking sign that said "In Heat." By the time our show was over, most everyone in the class was aching with laughter.

The official graduation ceremonies included the "hooding" of the vet school graduates. Certainly I was proud. There had been so many times when I'd thought I'd never see this moment. But what I remember the most about graduation was Myriah. I had always known that the minute I got out of school and was once again my own woman I would get a dog. I knew I wanted a yellow Labrador or a golden retriever, but before I could even begin to investigate the possibilities, a friend called saying he had had a golden retriever shipped to me. It was a female, which was what I'd wanted, and it would be arriving at the Columbus airport. Another friend, who also wanted a golden retriever, was getting my dog's littermate. Her dog was a male and he would be arriving along with mine.

We went to the airport together to pick up the puppies. Nothing gives me more intense pleasure and makes me feel more like a child than picking up a new pet. The pleasure of owning animals has never diminished for me. I couldn't wait to see my new puppy. Finally the arrival was announced and, after what seemed like endless waiting, we had our crate. We pried it open and out bounded the All-American adorable puppy. It was a beautiful beige with the wrinkled but noble face of the golden pup. Looking like a miniature teddy bear, it ran right up to me, squirming and licking. And then I noticed that it was a male. My dog, the female puppy, was sitting in the back corner of the crate. Forlorn and timid, she was such a picture of misery that my friend turned to me and said, "I'm sorry, Sally. That's the female."

My puppy was smaller than the male and she really didn't look like a golden. She was pretty, but she didn't have the loose skin on the face that gives the golden puppy its characteristic expression. She was also quiet and shy. Great, I thought, I wait years to get a puppy and then I get a dud. But it looked like I was stuck with her.

We went over to my friend's house where we gave the two pups the freedom of the backyard. As the male bounded about, full of charm and personality, I became increasingly depressed. I wanted so badly to keep him. I even named him: Molson, for Molson Golden beer. Finally I called the breeder. If there was another male in the litter, I would return the female, take Molson and give the new male to my friend, who had agreed to the plan. But there was no other male so I watched Myriah, as I'd finally named her, as she watched me and the rest of her new, frightening world.

The first few days with Myriah continued with no improvement in how either of us felt about our respective situations. Finally it was time to drive home to Mentor. I was glad to have Myriah with me, if only to take my mind off the sadness I felt at leaving OSU for the last time. I bundled her into the car along with an amazing amount of luggage and what I suppose could be called "collectibles" and we set off. The farther north we got, the more Myriah improved in her manner and personality. She relaxed and tried playing with my elbow as I drove, and she eventually settled down to sit beside me with great dignity. Now that we were alone together I began to see Myriah in a new light. I realized she had been overpowered by her domineering brother.She had been reasonably frightened of the whole experience of being taken from her mother and put in a crate and then on a plane to ride for hours to a new home. But she wasn't a wimp. She had her own special charm and personality and I just had to give her a chance to develop. It was a lesson to me and one that I remember whenever I see people who are disappointed or impatient with their puppies. If you get a dog while it's young, during its socialization period it will mold its personality to you. If you lavish attention on it while it's a pup, talk to it, introduce it to lots of people, show it affection, train it and give it tasks to do you'll be rewarded with a companion that will never disappoint you.

Myriah became my best friend and jogging partner in short order. Right from the beginning she went everywhere with me. Even today, as I write this, she's curled on the floor, resting after our morning run. If I glance over at her, she'll open one eye as if to ask me what I want, and if she senses that my attention is focused on her, she'll lift her tail once or twice to acknowledge me. She's a clown and a lady and if, when I first met her, she didn't have the instant appeal of her brother, it's been all the more pleasurable to watch Myriah come into her own as a dog of special character and charm. She's the best present I ever received.

MY FIRST JOB

CASTLE SHANNON

In the spring of my last year at OSU, as I had gone about the process of choosing a job—my first real job as a vet—my main goal had been to find a position that would allow me to continue to learn. For many vets four years of veterinary school is the sum total of their training. Once they graduate they can hang out a shingle and begin work. But most newly minted vets don't feel ready to open a practice, so it's common procedure to spend a few years with an experienced vet as a sort of apprenticeship before you buy into a practice or start one of your own.

I was determined that my graduation from OSU wouldn't be the end of my education. I wanted to get the best and the most experience I could. When I applied to practices and went for interviews, I looked first at the staff and the facilities and then at the hours and compensation. This wasn't noble or timid of me; it was just good sense. If I took a job at a practice that did only shots and spays, I figured that all the information currently filling my head would quickly rust with disuse. And I'd be bored. I wanted something to challenge me. The day might come when a small practice would give me the time to raise a family, but right now, for my first postgraduate job, I wanted as much variety as I could find. When I'd considered the job offers I'd had, Castle Shannon Animal Hospital seemed to be just what I was looking for. It offered good clinical

169

experience with a skilled staff, and it had a board-certified surgeon on staff. Many practices can't boast that and it meant that we'd be doing a good range of surgical cases. The hospital also had just hired a vet who'd completed a medical residency at Cornell. He'd no doubt be smart and experienced and I'd learn a lot from him. And, finally, Castle Shannon was in Pittsburgh, Pennsylvania, not too far from my friends, many of whom had stayed in Ohio.

Optimistic, enthusiastic, eager, willing, I arrived for my first day of work. It was a Tuesday in the beginning of July and one of those bright, clear early summer days that we all think of in the middle of February. I was elated as I drove through the suburbs of Pittsburgh and up to the low brick building with the "Castle Shannon Animal Hospital" sign near the curb. The hospital was large and airy, with four examining rooms and a cheerful reception area. I was so proud when I came in that first day. It was the first time I'd reported to work as a vet. I wondered if the clients already waiting with their cats and dogs could *tell* I was a vet. My boss, Dr. Evans, greeted me and invited me into his office for some coffee. After some pleasant chatter he leaned back in his chair and said, "Sally, we have some good and some bad news for you. The good news first. You'll be working only four days instead of the five days we'd agreed upon."

It's a measure of how anxious I was to get to work that in the first instant this didn't seem especially good news. I was eager to develop my own list of patients and start getting to know the dogs and cats of Pittsburgh and their owners. On the other hand, I'd well appreciate some free time. I had been living at a break-neck pace for over four years and a little relaxation would be nice. I could visit my relatives in Pittsburgh and drive the three hours to Mentor to see my family more often. After all the visits home I'd had to cancel because of vet school studies, I knew my parents would appreciate that. Letting my imagination run away, I began to think about how nice it would be to get to know the city and catch up on some movies and cultural events. The more I thought about it, the better this arrangement seemed.

"The bad news, Sally, is that you'll be working Saturday night emergency," Dr. Evans said, his eyes searching my face for a reaction. I was busy trying to figure out the implications of this change of schedule. No one really likes to work an overnight emergency shift because it means working all through the night and because it can be so unpredictable: for hours you'll have little to do and then there's a landslide. I also quickly realized that the extra day off that I already had so many wonderful plans for would probably be taken up with sleep as I'd be coming off a twenty-four-hour shift. But I knew the drawbacks of all-night emergency shifts only by reputation. I might find that Saturday night had its advantages. After all, as I'd be the only doctor there, I'd be in charge and that was a heady thought. Was it possible I might even come to enjoy Saturday night? My optimism got the best of me and I assured Dr. Evans that his plan would work out fine. We chatted for a few more minutes and I went off to begin my first day of work.

As I didn't yet have clients of my own, I spent most of those first few days at Castle Shannon handling clients who hadn't requested a specific vet, learning my way around the hospital and doing routine tasks for the other vets. Even though I wasn't fully plugged into the system, I found the pace frantic. It was during that summer that parvo became a menace to the dog population of the East Coast, and the parvo epidemic completely changed the atmosphere at Castle Shannon and sometimes made it seem more a bunker against an invading enemy than a peaceful animal hospital.

Parvo is a virus that particularly attacks puppies and older dogs, but any dog can catch it. It acts quickly: an animal can be fine one night, slightly listless the next morning and deathly sick by the same evening. Stricken dogs usually become feverish, anorexic, lethargic and dehydrated and they develop vomiting and bloody diarrhea.

Because parvo was a new disease and because there was such an epidemic of it, people were justifiably frightened. Puppies, in particular, were dying by the dozens. Pet owners were rushing in to Castle Shannon to get their dogs inoculated against parvo but we didn't have enough vaccine to go around. The demand was outrageous and we were in the painful position of trying to allot the supply of vaccine as best we could on a first-come-first-served basis. It seemed the waiting room was always jammed and even the parking lot was full of the people who couldn't fit inside. There were so many people that every day when we ran out of vaccine we'd have to turn them away. And we'd only take cases by appointment. People would often call asking for the parvo vaccine and we'd have to tell them that we were booked up, with all available vaccine allocated for the next week. Those same people would come in the middle of the night to the emergency service with a dog that had a slight cough or an ear infection and after we'd treated the minor problem they'd say, "While I'm here I might as well get her that vaccination for that parvo disease." Suddenly the reason for the middle-of-the-night visit would become clear. But I couldn't blame these people. I understood just how they felt.

Myriah was only ten weeks old when we arrived at Castle Shannon. Even in the short time I'd had her, she'd become so much a part of my life that I couldn't imagine things without her. She was and is a special dog. And in those early days in Pittsburgh she was at her cutest, teddy-bear best. The specter of parvo, the experience of watching other people's puppies die of the disease, made Myriah seem all the more precious to me. Because I was working long shifts—from 8 A.M. to 10 P.M.—I couldn't leave her home alone, so every day she came to the hospital with me. This meant that Myriah was being exposed to parvo every single day, and even though I'd vaccinated her she may not have built up enough immunity. Poor Myriah was watched more carefully than any puppy ever had been. The slightest variation in her behavior was calibrated.

Myriah never did get parvo and it was at Castle Shannon that she was broken into the pattern of coming to work with me and immediately adjusting to a multitude of strange dogs, cats, birds and other animals.

No matter what your profession, the big difference between learning and doing is emergencies. They land on you without warning and call upon not only your best skills but also your best character. You have to think with all possible speed and act with careful deliberation. It's a challenge and one that you can never really be prepared for. In vet school we worked with all manner of sick animals. We treated acute and chronic illness and we performed surgery. But nothing but a real emergency with an animal dying before your eyes and an owner hysterical with grief and a sudden shortage of help can crack the shell of the innocence of your chosen career.

I'd had only two days of work at Castle Shannon before I arrived for my first all-night emergency shift. It was 8 A.M. on Saturday and I was feeling as fresh and energetic as a colt on a May morning. In two days of work I'd gotten to know my way around the hospital a bit—at least I knew where to look for most of the supplies—and I was beginning to get to know the people. Little did I dream that twenty-four hours later my initial poise and confidence would seem a mockery.

The first thing I learned on emergency duty was there was no routine or schedule to the twenty-four hours. Things were handled on a sort of triage system: the most critical cases got looked at first and the goal was simply to stabilize the animal. Usually I treated any emergencies that came in from five o'clock in the afternoon to one in the morning and then at 1 A.M., or as soon as I had a minute, I began surgeries. Because there was no scheduled surgery on Saturday, any surgery cases that came in on an emergency basis were handled as soon as I was free from stabilizing the more desperate emergency cases. On the average night I would be doing surgeries from the wee hours of the morning until about 5 A.M. when new emergencies began to roll in again. It's a measure of my youth and inexperience that this schedule seemed more a challenge than a wheel upon which the foolishness of the new veterinarian would be broken.

The first hour of my shift was calm. I treated two or three animals who arrived as if scheduled in about twenty-minute intervals. This was going to be a piece of cake, I thought. And then it began. The earthquake. The landslide. The tempest. I soon learned that we were about the only animal clinic in Pittsburgh that stayed open through the night. I was the one in charge—the only vet at work in the south side of the city I realized—and with the help of a technician I had to somehow get through the night. My heart began to race.

It was hard to believe that so many different emergencies could arrive at the hospital in a single night. I had blocked cats, hit-by-cars, kidney failures, cut paw pads, antifreeze poisonings and a number of new parvo cases. I was in the middle of unblocking a cat when I got a call from downstairs: one of the in-house patients, an epileptic collie, had gone into *status epilepticus*—a continual epileptic seizure. He needed to be brought out of it immediately or he would die. In this prolonged seizure the temperature elevates to 107 and all the sugar in the body is burned up. If oxygen doesn't get to the brain the animal will die quickly. I left my cat and rushed downstairs with my heart pounding. As I ran I was reviewing how I'd treat the seizure. I knew that I'd have to get some Valium into him right away in order to relax him and stop the seizure.

When I arrived in the back ward I found a thrashing, salivating, jaw-chomping dog and a technician valiantly trying to restrain him. A dog in a seizure can be dangerous because he has enormous strength and can inflict a serious bite. I grabbed a needle and tried to get it into the cephalic vein. The technician who was holding the dog was doing a magnificent job, but with all the movement, and despite repeated stabs, I simply couldn't get the needle into the thrashing leg's vein. It seemed like hours, but after a few futile stabs, a "tomato" emerged. A "tomato," or technically a hematoma, is a lump formed when blood seeps out of the vein. A hematoma heals in a day or two and doesn't harm the animal but it's sloppy technique and makes it impossible to find the vein in that area. I was sweating and desperate. I had to get that dog's vein or he could die. The technician, seeing my distress, took the needle from me and while I threw myself on the dog she inserted it with her first try. I almost wept with relief.

I was drenched with sweat by the time I got the Valium into the dog. We waited a few minutes but nothing happened. The dog was still in seizure. I knew that I'd have to try some phenobarbital next but I didn't know where it was kept. Because it's such a strong, addictive drug only the vets knew where it was and the technician couldn't help me. Meanwhile, as I made a frantic search through the hastily unlocked cabinets, trying to breathe deeply, trying to stay calm, trying not to spill medications in my frantic search, the dog continued his seizure. I knew he couldn't last long.

Desperate, I grabbed the phone and called Dr. Evans. I'm sure my efforts to sound composed and in control were futile. But Dr. Evans was calm and reassuring. I told him I had a dog in a prolonged seizure that wasn't responding to Valium. He confirmed that phenobarbital would be the next step and he told me where to find it. Listening to a rational, authoritative voice was like a quick belt of brandy. Calmed, I felt my confidence return.

Just as I hung up the phone, I heard the page calling me from upstairs. There was a cockatiel upstairs who had flown into a window and now had a bleeding beak and they couldn't get the bleeding to stop. Birds can't afford to lose much blood; heavy, unstopped bleeding is soon fatal. Oh, Lord, I thought, my heart racing again, a bird emergency. I'd had one course on birds and liked them but I'd had little experience handling them.

My first night on the job was beginning to seem like "I Love Lucy Goes to the Animal Hospital." In my second hour of work I had a blocked cat, a dog in a life-threatening seizure and a cockatiel with a bleeding beak that needed immediate attention and who knew what other serious if less critical emergencies were lurking upstairs. No class I'd taken, no experience in an office, nothing I'd read or heard had prepared me for this. I kept repeating to myself over and over: *"Stay calm. Stay calm."* Eventually the words became meaningless but the mindless repetition helped me.

I quickly found the phenobarbital and got it into the dog. I could feel his body relax under my hand and my relief was indescribable. His pulse was weak but he was alive and would probably survive.

The pace was nonstop. I dealt with the cat, got the bird to stop bleeding and went on to cope with an astonishing number of sick and injured animals. I have since learned that emergency clinics vary by geography and weather. In New York people will bring an animal into the emergency clinic in the middle of the night with a problem that's existed for weeks. Perhaps the level of insomnia in Manhattan has something to do with that. In North Carolina, animals were often bitten by snakes. In very bad weather, no matter where you are, the number of emergency cases usually goes down, perhaps because animals are inside where they are safe from cars and each other. In summer, pets in the outdoors are vulnerable to many dangers as well as the weather itself, which induces many cases of heat stroke in pets who are left in cars or exercised too much. A beautiful summer day will send pets to the emergency hospital with parvo, lacerations, cut paw pads and the inevitable HBC's. On that July night in Pittsburgh there seemed to be a convergence of factors that made for an unending stream of bona fide animal emergencies.

At 1 A.M. that Sunday morning, exhausted by worry as much as the frantic activity, I began my surgery cases. Until five I stitched lacerations, drained abscesses, sutured paw pads and even anesthetized a dog to remove a fishhook. By the time

I had finished with the surgeries, the second round of emergencies started to trickle in. I had lost all sense of time. I had always been working and always would be. Sleep and meals and normal conversations with other human beings were things of the past. I had become a machine that wanted to know symptoms, conditions and history as quickly as possible and then I wanted to move immediately to solve the problem before the next case came in.

At last it was 8 A.M. and the shift was over. But I couldn't yet leave. I had to finish up with the cases that had come in up until eight and then I had to make phone calls. It was important to call the owners of the pets I'd treated to give them an update on their animal's condition. I'd quickly learned that the worst thing you can do to a pet owner is keep them in the dark. Sometimes you have so much to do and so little time and your energy is so concentrated on the animal itself that you forget that at home someone is worried sick over their pet's fate. So I took a few more minutes, a little more time on automatic pilot, and reported on the status of my patients. It's a simple task and it can be emotionally draining sometimes, but that morning, exhausted by the twenty-four hours I'd been through, I felt almost relaxed as I gave clients the eagerly awaited news. Then I was finished.

As I made my way home the city was beginning to stir. I watched people heading for church and people heading home with the Sunday papers under their arms, probably looking forward to a leisurely summer afternoon. I was numb. As I drew the shades and climbed into bed my mind was still racing. Emergency medicine is certainly a different world from routine care. It takes guts. You have full responsibility for all the animals in the hospital. You're forced to take charge and make quick decisions and act on them. Many of the cases are a matter of life and death. During the day the board-certified surgeon would handle a difficult surgery case because he has more experience and therefore the animal has a better chance. But at night on emergency you do it yourself as well as you

can even if you've never done it before. You do your best and
hope for the best.

After the shock of my first night on emergency wore off,
I discovered I loved it. Not only that, it was good for me.
There is an element to performing surgeries and doctoring
animals that goes beyond knowledge and depends on physical
grace and precision. Like a great fastball or a heroic long jump,
your performance can depend on some precise, mysterious
balance of mind and body. When you're on emergencies, working fast and hard, you burn out all the indecision and false
impulses. You can find that you're at your best and your
confidence is soaring. Time and again that happened to me
and it spilled over into my daily work. Not only was I per-
fecting my skills, but I was adopting a confident mental posture that was making me a good vet.

So as it turned out, Dr. Evans did have some bad news for
me and some good news. He just had them mixed up. The
good news wasn't the shorter work week. As it turned out,
because of my Saturday night shift and another all-night emergency shift every other Tuesday, I was back to my usual frantic
pace. I wasn't going to have any leisure. I wasn't going to see
my family. I wasn't going to get to know the city. But the
good news was that I had Saturday night emergencies—my
first opportunity to take real responsibility for so many different cases. One animal after another came in in desperate
straits and most of them left in a few days good as new. The
satisfaction I took from that was enormous. Like a baby thrown
into the water, I was learning to swim.

THE ORANGE CLOTHESPIN

My schedule at Castle Shannon included surgery slots two
mornings a week. My first case was a Pomeranian. She was

about one year old and was in for a spay. There were still so many unfamiliar things to cope with. But a surgery would be like coming home. I knew I'd feel at ease and in control once I began. I entered the surgery room to find the little Pomeranian bouncing across the table. She was a hyperactive dog and I could see that I'd need some help restraining her. There were two technicians to help me. They had drawn up the correct dosage of Surital, the short-acting anesthetic, which I would use to relax the dog so she could be intubated for inhalation anesthesia.

I had met the two technicians and liked them very much. Still, there is a sort of inevitable nervousness to performing for the first time before an experienced audience. But they relaxed me with a few jokes as they struggled to hold down the little dog. It's not overkill to have two healthy humans hold down a ten-pound Pomeranian because a very excited dog who's determined to postpone her surgery to another, more agreeable time is a wily and resourceful opponent. It was experienced human strength versus determined dog will as we tried to get her still enough to get the needle into her vein. When at last she was immobile for a few seconds, I grabbed the little paw and inserted the needle in the vein on the front of her leg on the first try. I was pleased the technicians didn't have to witness me making jab after jab. Things were off to a good start.

As the technicians continued to restrain the dog, I slowly injected the anesthetic. I had administered about three quarters of the dosage when, within a matter of seconds, the little dog went into respiratory arrest, then cardiac arrest. We attempted cardiopulmonary resuscitation, but to no avail. I stood over the small body in shock, oblivious for the first time that morning of my audience.

The poor dog died so quickly I could hardly believe it had happened. As the technicians began to pat my arm and reassure me that I had done the right thing and that the dosage was correct and that this sort of thing can happen to anyone,

I stood there with tears in my eyes, all my energies focused on not crying. I wanted nothing more than to disappear from the spot, to be removed like Dorothy from Kansas to another place where no one knew me and where I could begin a new life. Two awful things had happened: first and worst was that a dog, a dog that had been happy and healthy only minutes before, had died under my care. Second, in my first surgery of my first real job, I'd been a failure. I had been confident I was a good surgeon and would get even better with practice. But these people at Castle Shannon knew nothing about me. And now they'd seen me kill my first patient. What would we tell the dog's owner? Would I ever be able to salvage my reputation?

Inevitably in the course of a career as a veterinarian you will lose some cases. There are occasionally cases of dogs and cats that die on the operating table from an anesthetic because it was impossible to predict their drug tolerance. Dosages are given by weight but there are some contradictions to the rules. Some large dogs like Irish wolfhounds should get far less anesthetic or medication per pound of body weight than you would think if you extrapolated from the dosages given to medium-size dogs. Worst of all, there are occasionally dogs of any size or breed whose systems seem unable to tolerate much anesthetic at all and with them you never know in advance what their reaction to a drug will be. Every animal metabolizes an anesthetic differently. In pets six years or older we routinely do blood work to check out liver and kidney function to be sure they can handle the anesthetic. But of course the Pomeranian was only one and there was no indication she couldn't handle the anesthetic.

All of this I knew, but it was no consolation that morning. Left to my own devices, I would have put my head down on the table and wept. But the technicians wouldn't allow it. They kept saying, "Don't let it get you down. It could have happened to anyone. You didn't do a thing wrong." Within minutes they had me moving over to another table where a cat had been knocked down already and was waiting to be declawed. I successfully performed that surgery and one or two other routine ones and was finished with my surgical cases for that first day.

Immediately after I finished my surgical shift I went to Dr. Bredel, the vet who worked on my team, and described what had happened on my first case. He was understanding, as he had seen that sort of thing happen before, but naturally he wasn't pleased. He knew there was nothing I could have done but that's little comfort when a vet has to call an owner and tell them their pet has died. Because the Pomeranian had been someone else's case when she came in, another vet handled this painful job of informing the owner.

Despite the dismal beginning to my day, I still had hours of work to face. Things were so busy, and I was soon so involved giving parvo shots and treating routine cases, that the morning seemed to recede in time. By dinnertime I was working with enthusiasm and had placed the morning's experience in the back of my mind.

Castle Shannon Animal Hospital has a particular way of identifying animals' charts for the vets who work there: "the Clothespin System." There is a rack and as the animals come in, if a client requests a certain vet, their charts are put on the rack marked with a colored clothespin. Each vet is assigned a different color for their clothespins. The system saved time because a vet could breeze through the reception area and quickly see if she had any cases waiting for her. My color was orange. As I'd only been at the hospital for two days and didn't have any clients request me yet, I hadn't had a clothespin turn up for me. Through the course of the day I'd take new patients who came in and didn't already have a relationship with another vet. I'd walk through the reception area and see red clothespins and yellow. Dr. Bredel had black clothespins and there were always a sea of black pins. His wife, who also worked there as a vet, was blue, and she always had a good collection of pins too. But so far, no orange clothespins.

That night at about six-thirty and just before clinics, I walked through the reception room. There was an orange clothespin! Someone had requested me. I was thrilled. I grabbed the chart and, grinning at the girl at the front desk, I said, "Wow! Somebody asked for me. This isn't a mistake is it? It should be an orange clothespin, right?" The receptionist was looking very sober and I couldn't understand why she wasn't sharing my pleasure. I soon found out. "Sally," she said, "it's the owner of the Pomeranian."

My first clothespin—the first client to request me at my first job—was the owner of the Pomeranian who had died at my hands that morning. It had seemed so long ago, and now, suddenly, it was all as fresh as if it had just happened. What was I going to say to this woman? Dr. Bredel appeared at my side and told me not to worry, that he was going to talk with her and explain that it was an unpredictable anesthetic reaction. I waited outside his office, more nervous than I'd been before any exam in all my years of veterinary training. Nothing had prepared me for this.

When Dr. Bredel ushered me into the room I was facing a grim middle-aged woman. "Dr. Bredel has explained things to me, Dr. Haddock, but I still want to know exactly what happened from someone who was there." Was there a strong emphasis on her last few words or was I imagining things?

"I can't tell you how sorry I am about your dog. I have a dog, too, a puppy, and I can imagine how difficult this must be for you. But there was no way I could have predicted that your dog would react that way to the anesthetic." The woman was upset but reasonable. She wanted to know about skin testing or other ways of allergic testing that could have prevented her dog's death. I made the best explanation I could to her, but I was really too upset myself to make a precise medical analysis of the situation. Still my concern and distress must have helped convince the woman her dog's death wasn't due to carelessness.

It was a good thing I had hours of work yet to do that night because I think if I had gone home alone and spent the evening reliving my first day of surgery, it might have been my last. It was becoming clear to me that veterinary medicine was only partly the care of animals. It was also dealing with people, sometimes under very difficult circumstances.

"LET'S ROCK 'ER"

When I think about putting pets to sleep—unquestionably the most difficult part of my job—I think about Sunshine, the yellow Lab.

Sunshine became my patient on an autumn day, crisp and clear, when the leaves at Castle Shannon were just beginning to turn color. I was no longer a student. It was the first autumn of my life that wasn't being spent getting ready for school and I felt just a bit nostalgic for all my falls at OSU and the swarms of good friends who'd filled my days. But I was enjoying my work and developing a clientele of my own. I was experiencing a very different and new kind of pleasure.

On this particular autumn morning a group came into my examining room that looked like they had just stepped out of a magazine ad. The mother was pretty and blond. Holding one of her hands was a little boy of about five years with the same blond hair and a gap-toothed smile. A little girl about eight years old and as pretty as her mother followed, holding a leash, and last but not least came the reason for the visit. Sunshine was a handsome yellow Labrador retriever. She was about ten years old and, despite the fact that she looked perfectly healthy, the family had noticed that she was having difficulty urinating. After taking a history and Sunshine, I realized I would have to do an extensive work-up on her to discover the problem. The family would have to leave her at the hospital. Rarely have I seen a more touching parting, as the little boy threw his arms around Sunshine's neck and the girl, crying, kissed her big wet nose. I kept reminding the kids that Sunshine was going to be with me for only a couple of days, but that did little to reassure them. Only Sunshine seemed unaffected by anxiety.

Over the course of the next two days we did a series of tests and discovered that Sunshine was suffering from *granulomatous urethritis*. That's a disease that afflicts older female dogs and it's not terribly uncommon. The disease causes a thickening of the urethra, the tube that leaves the bladder and through which the dog passes urine. As the tube thickens it closes and the dog finds it more and more difficult to urinate. Unfortunately *granulomatous urethritis* is not curable. We can pass a catheter through the urethra and the dog will be able to urinate through it, but if the catheter is removed, the urethra will usually obstruct again.

I called the mother with the bad news. I told her the prognosis for Sunshine was poor. There was only one option and it was fairly daunting. We could catheterize the dog, leaving the catheter in place. A plug is put in the end of the catheter and every day, three or four times a day, the owner takes the dog out, unplugs it and lets it urinate. Though there is a chance of infections with this method and Sunshine would have to stay on antibiotics, the dog is usually comfortable with this arrangement. It's the owners who suffer the inconvenience and sometimes neighbors need to be taken into confidence so they don't become suspicious about the unorthodox dog-walking routine. With their hectic household the mother felt that option wasn't really practical. She decided to come in with the children to say good-bye to Sunshine before she was put to sleep.

This was a visit I wasn't looking forward to. Any vet would have difficulty with the situation, but for me it was even worse because usually, when I have to watch people go through this sort of thing, I begin to cry as well. No matter how many times I've been through it, it never fails to touch me.

The next day the family trooped in again. The girl had on a pretty dress and the little boy's hair was freshly combed.

Sunshine's farewell was going to be a formal event. The girl was holding Sunshine's leash while the boy carried a pink rubber bone—Sunshine's favorite toy. When I brought the dog into the examining room, the children rushed her. Sunshine was convulsed with pleasure at seeing her family again and was no doubt eager to jump into the car and forget this unpleasant interlude of strange people and irritating tests.

The little boy eventually looked up at me, a tear sliding down his cheek, and asked what would happen to Sunshine. I glanced at the mother and she nodded. I told the children she was very sick and would never get better. Because she would be unhappy and in pain if we didn't do anything, I was going to give her a special drug that would put her to sleep forever. She wouldn't feel anything and she'd only remember the happy times she'd had with them. Then, maybe after a few months, they could get another dog. I didn't know if the mother had had this in mind but I figured the idea of a new pet would at least partly take the children's minds off Sunshine.

The little boy looked dubious. With his arm still around Sunshine's neck and his face next to hers he asked me, "What will she be like when she's dead?" "Well," I said, "her spirit will be gone to doggie heaven and her body will be left behind. She'll be still and quiet like a rock." By this time my eyes were wet and I was swallowing hard. The dog seemed so healthy, indeed was wagging her tail fiercely as she tried to lick the girl and boy simultaneously.

"There is one more thing," I said, "one thing that you could do but it would be very difficult and it might not be the best thing for Sunshine." I caught the mother's eye to see if she objected to my bringing up the catheterization option. She nodded. "We could put a tube in Sunshine to help her pass her urine. But if I did that you'd all have to help her every day."

"What do you think, Susie?" the mother said to the little girl. Both children were silent, lost in thought.

Finally the little boy piped up. "No," he said, "let's rock
'er."

My jaw dropped. I'll never know if the children were simply
reflecting the discussion the mother told me they'd had at
home where they decided that the best thing for Sunshine was
to let her go to heaven or if the idea of Sunshine being quiet
as a rock was so fascinating they couldn't resist opting for it.
The clinic aide who was in the room began to laugh. I began
to laugh and soon everyone was laughing. The laughter was
a welcome release of tension, and when it came time to say
good-bye to Sunshine, I was able to proceed with a stiff upper
lip. Sunshine was "rocked" and I got a new insight into the
forthright curiosity of children.

THE BITE

There is one particular problem that vets have with their
patients that human doctors generally avoid—biting. It isn't
always easy to restrain an unfriendly animal while you examine it, give it injections or medicate it. Some dogs are under-
standably nervous or frightened, but in many cases the problem
originates with the owner. I've seen many dog owners who
were afraid of their pets. They somehow managed to get a
dominant dog and the dog, a pack animal to begin with, soon
realizes it can call the shots. These dogs sometimes get so
inflated with their sense of power they will bite if crossed.
On many occasions I've had trouble trying to muzzle a dog
in order to treat it, and when I've asked the owner to help,
they've refused. They're simply afraid.

Worse than the accidental mismatching of a dominant dog
and a docile human is the dog trained to attack for sport rather
than business. It's one thing for a dog to be professionally
trained as a guard or police dog. It's quite another for an
amateur to train his dog to attack for "fun." I think some

misguided people take a twisted pride in owning an animal that will attack others and will accept only them as the master. Certainly there's a sense of power involved. But these animals are really a hazard to vets as well as to the general public if they aren't controlled.

I always tell people who own vicious dogs that they're living with a time bomb. You never know when such a dog will turn on you and bite, and you never know if the victim will be a child who could suffer massive injuries or even death. How would they feel if their dog took a child's life? I remind them that today, when people sue over the most trivial matters, a biting dog is an invitation to financial disaster for them as well. My advice to owners of such dogs, dogs that they can't control, is to find them a home with someone who can or to have them put humanely to sleep. There are so many good, intelligent, homeless dogs available there's no reason to own one that is a liability to yourself and to others.

One of the most unusual cases of an attack dog I ever saw was while I was working at Castle Shannon Animal Hospital. One day a man came in with a German shepherd. The dog needed to have his ears cleaned out and he was due for a vaccination. The animal was friendly and good-natured and barely flinched as I worked on his ears. When I'd finished, the dog's owner told me he had trained the dog himself. Without any professional help, using books that he'd found on the subject, he trained the dog to obey him completely. I congratulated him on his achievement but in the back of my mind I wondered why he seemed so particularly proud of his dog training as it's not so uncommon. Then he asked me if I'd like to see his dog perform. Certainly I would. The dog was sitting calmly on the table. I was scratching his neck and he was licking my hand. The owner asked me to move to the other side of the examining room. I was ready to watch the dog sit on his hind legs or count or even sing—accomplishments that could make any trainer especially proud. Instead, after the owner leaned down and put his head right beside his dog's, the animal was transformed from a docile pet into a raging beast. He was barking and snarling and doing his best to strain his leash to the breaking point so he could wreak havoc on my person. The smile on my face became a grimace.

How does one react to a dog that clearly would savor ripping out your throat? At another command that was invisible to me, the dog again became his sweet, agreeable self. I was speechless but the owner was only too happy to explain to me that he'd trained the dog to attack on a whispered command. A shouted command would get no response, but a soft "attack" whispered into the dog's ears had him at the ready. The man claimed he had developed this method because he never wanted the dog to attack except to defend the owner's life and this way only he knew the dog's secret trigger, which would presumably shock and disarm an enemy. Unusual as this man's training was, and alarming as I found it when it was demonstrated, I still think that the man was a responsible dog owner because he had complete control over his animal. Control is always the key.

It was while working at Castle Shannon that I got the worst and most frightening bite of my career thus far. A terrier-cross dog had come in to be treated for a skin problem. Certain breeds have a greater tendency to bite than others. No matter what owners or breed fanciers will say, vets get their experience on the front line. In my opinion, German shepherds, Chihuahuas, chow chows and sharpeis are among the most frequent biters. I've encountered dogs of these breeds that are friendly and well behaved and I'd be the last one to condemn a breed because of particular problems I've seen, but you can't ignore your personal experience.

I examined the dog, told the owner how we were going to treat the skin problem. It was flea bite allergy. Although we found only a couple of fleas and associated flea dirt, the bite of one flea can set off an allergic reaction to the flea's saliva. The saliva causes the dog to start biting and scratching and exacerbates the problem. The cure is cortisone and flea control. I gave the dog his shots for the skin problem, his vaccinations and was ready to wind up the visit. But before I lifted him from the table, the owner asked me if I would clip the terrier's dewclaws. The dewclaw is a vestigial toe that is on the inside edge of a leg, usually a few inches above the foot. Not all dogs have them but many large breeds do; indeed the Great Pyrenees have two. Many dogs have their dewclaws removed a few days after they're born, especially if they're working dogs and the dewclaw would be liable to injury. Dogs that never need their other nails clipped will sometimes need the dewclaw nail clipped. That's because constant scratching on pavement usually keeps a dog's nails short, but as the dewclaw doesn't touch the ground it never comes in contact with the most popular doggie nail file. In fact, city dogs, because they're always working on their nails, rarely need them cut, but country dogs, who have no access to concrete, blacktop and cement, must depend on artificial manicures.

At any rate this terrier needed his dewclaw nails clipped, so I bent and, with the clipper, trimmed one and then went for the other. The terrier wheeled around and lunged for me. The force of his attack threw me against the wall. The most curious aspect of being the victim of such a violent assault is that immediately afterward you're not really sure of what has happened. Only after a few minutes go by do you begin to appreciate your condition. I stood against the wall and lifted my hand to my head. I felt certain that was where the dog had struck. I was feeling for blood. The owner of the dog grabbed the animal and apologized and, as I told him that it was nothing to worry about, I saw the blood on my hand. I knew I should take a look at my forehead so I went into the hall where another vet named Sue saw me, grabbed an ice pack and pressed it to my head.

A few minutes went by with me sitting in a chair and Sue holding the ice pack to my head. I felt sheepish and hoped no clients would come by and witness this curious scene. Finally, Sue, lifting the ice pack, said she wanted to see what the wound looked like. Sue's mouth dropped open and her eyes widened. As her nose was inches from mine, it was hard for me to feign indifference to her reaction. "Remind me never to play poker with you, Sue," I said. "Oh, it's just a puncture wound," she replied, trying to recover. "A puncture wound made by a pencil or a telephone pole?" I wondered. I headed into the bathroom to take a look at it. Sue grabbed my arm. "Are you sure you want to look? Maybe we should just go to the hospital and have it taken care of?"

I'm not a squeamish person. In fact, after I got that finger shortened in a door hinge in college, the emergency room staff at the hospital told me they'd never seen such a relaxed, slightly dismembered person. So I really wasn't afraid of looking at my puncture wound. But I should have been. I had a quarter-sized hole above my eye, half my eyebrow was missing and the muscle above my eye was half-gone. I looked like something out of a Frankenstein movie.

A technician drove me to the hospital and within a few minutes I was in the emergency room. A plastic surgeon was called and fortunately was there in just a few minutes. A nurse asked me if I had the missing skin piece and I explained to her that she'd have to discuss that with a terrier who could be recognized by one of his dewclaws, which was slightly longer than the other. Nonetheless, they called the clinic to see if there was any skin lying around the examing room but none ever turned up. The plastic surgeon went to work within seconds of his arrival. As I was under a local anesthetic, I could talk with him and it was a good thing too. He at first wanted to graft some skin from my thigh to my forehead. "You can't do that," I told him. "I was riding a mechanical bull yesterday and I have bruises all over my legs. If there's one thing worse than a hole in your head, it's a bruised hole." He agreed that it could be bad for his business to start grafting bruises.

As it turned out, the surgeon decided to forget the graft and stitch the hole together. It's easier to close an oval or linear wound than a round one because the edges are closer together. When you close a circular wound you invariably have some puckering of the edges. Well, he did a nice job of sewing me up and after a few follow-up treatments I was almost back to normal.

In my opinion the worst part of this story is the aftermath. It turns out that the woman who owned the dog had told her husband to warn the vet that the dog had snapped at people before. He hadn't bothered. Moreover, when the time came for me to go to another plastic surgeon to get a second opinion, the owners of the dog wouldn't help out with the medical costs that weren't covered by workman's comp—costs I would have to shoulder myself. Many people urged me to sue them, at least for my costs, but I didn't have the heart for it. Ultimately the incident damaged my faith in human nature without affecting my warm feelings toward dogs, including terriers. But these days I'm more careful both about riding mechanical bulls and clipping dewclaws.

SANFORD'S CHRISTMAS

My first Christmas of my first real job on my first year out of vet school was turning out to be a major disappointment. It was being ruined by the very stuff of Christmas: snow.

The holiday that year fell on a Thursday and I'd been planning long in advance for a family celebration in Mentor. My brother and of course my parents would be there and I hadn't been home to see them in so long it was going to be a special treat to catch up with them and fill them in on my experiences at Castle Shannon. I'd also finally have a chance to visit with friends from high school whom I hadn't seen in years. I'd been working fourteen-hour days and one twenty-four-hour shift on Saturday so it would be wonderful to have a day of peace and relaxation highlighted by family and good friends. It was a day to look forward to.

My plan was to leave Pittsburgh on Wednesday, have all of Thursday—Christmas Day—at home. On Friday morning, full of good food, I'd drive the three hours back to the animal hospital, arriving by noon, which is when I had to be back at work. Two things conspired against this plan. First, as low woman on the totem pole at work, I was selected at the last minute to be at work not at noon on Friday but at 8 A.M. This meant that I'd have to leave Mentor by around four in the morning. It would be a grueling drive followed by a full day of work but I'd certainly experienced worse so I continued wrapping my presents and hoping my mother would make two kinds of pie and that there'd be enough left over for me to spirit a few slices back to Pennsylvania.

On Wednesday evening my dreams of a white Christmas turned into a typical snow-belt nightmare and the second monkey wrench landed right in the middle of my plans. We were having a blizzard. Since those days I've lived in New York, where a few inches of snow immobilizes the population and everyone gets very proud about laying down arms for a few hours while they pull together like "real New Yorkers." Well, Ohio snow is a different matter altogether. It's not fun, especially if you have driving to do; it doesn't go away the next day; and it can be life-threatening. Once when I was in vet school I was driving during an Ohio blizzard and I was lucky to live to tell the tale. So when this Christmas blizzard began, my hopes of getting to Mentor and, worse, back to work by 8 A.M. on Friday began to dissolve. I didn't even have someone to drive with, someone to sing camp songs with as we slipped into frozen oblivion in a drift beside Route 306. I decided I didn't want to die alone and so I was therefore going to have the loneliest Christmas of my life there in Pittsburgh. I called my parents, packed away my presents and settled in to feel as sorry for myself as I possibly could.

There is nothing like a few hours of self-pity to bore the pants off you, so by Christmas Eve I decided to snap myself out of my misery. I figured the best place to cheer up would be work. I called the hospital and told the vet on duty that as I couldn't go home, I'd be happy to take over from whoever had the shift on Christmas Day. There was much jubilation on the phone and I got to feel like a heroine for at least a few minutes. I imagined myself spending Christmas performing emergency surgeries on a host of critical animals and saving lives left and right. What a noble gesture! What a noble person! And then the vet rang off saying that I could expect a very quiet day. He was at the moment alone with one dog recovering from surgery, a cat with an abscess and Sanford. Well, I wouldn't be a hero, I'd just be spending a quiet Christmas with Sanford. That brought me back down to earth. I called my family, wished them a Merry Christmas and fell into bed. But instead of falling asleep I lay awake thinking about Sanford.

Sanford was a black Labrador puppy who'd come to us at about Thanksgiving time. He was an HBC—"hit by car"—and his owners rushed in to the hospital carrying him in their arms. Sanford was owned by a young couple and they were terribly worried about him. They'd had him just a short time but they were already very attached to him. He was only a few months old and he'd run after a squirrel or a ball or something that had caught his attention out of their yard and into the street. I'll never forget how struck I was by the eyes of the wife. They had such care and concern in them. Just one look at her face told me that Sanford was a lucky dog.

It turned out that there was another reason for the worry on their faces. They were concerned about the cost of treating Sanford. Many people won't come right out and say that they can't afford to treat their animals. Especially because they can hardly bear to admit it to themselves. But people do give signals when they're worried about costs and a vet soon learns to recognize them. Sanford's owners checked in advance how much every procedure would cost and I quickly realized that though they loved their dog, they didn't have a lot of money to spend on expensive medical treatment. Whatever was wrong with him, I decided I'd take the most conservative approach possible and keep their bill down as much as I could.

I examined Sanford and discovered that he'd been lucky. He had some abrasions but an X ray revealed no broken bones and no internal injuries. I treated his cuts and released him to two very happy people.

Unfortunately, that wasn't the end of Sanford's story. A few weeks later he reappeared. He was having trouble breathing. I X-rayed him again and quickly saw what the problem was. Sanford had a diaphragmatic hernia. When he was hit by the car, a tiny tear probably occurred in his diaphragm. It was too small at that point to be a problem, but since then Sanford had been busy running and jumping and the stress of all this activity had taken its toll: the tiny tear had enlarged and now portions of his liver and his intestine were protruding through the tear into his chest. That's why he was having trouble breathing. Because there were all those extra organs in his chest cavity, Sanford couldn't inflate his lungs sufficiently.

Sanford would have to be operated on. While some dogs can live for a long time with an untreated diaphragmatic hernia, the more common result is death from a related complication. Eventually the hernia could cut off circulation in the intestine or compromise the liver or ultimately cause a fatal toxic condition or suffocate the pet. With a young, active puppy who was already having difficulty breathing, there didn't seem to be any hope for him without surgery.

Before I told the couple about the results of the X ray, I consulted my boss. I explained to him that I didn't think Sanford's owners could afford the surgery. I'd never operated on a diaphragmatic hernia because it was a complicated procedure usually performed by an experienced surgeon. But I knew how to do the surgery. I suggested that Dr. Evans, the owner of the hospital, allow me to operate on Sanford for a reduced fee. I would get the experience and the couple would save money. Dr. Evans agreed.

I told the couple my diagnosis and explained the costs. I told them that with the surgery, the hernia could be completely cleared up and, barring complications, if there were no severe adhesions of intestines, etc., in the chest, there was almost no chance it would cause any future trouble. The estimate for the total bill was around $200, but as the surgery would be done for cost they would be saving a considerable amount of money.

Both the husband and wife reacted simultaneously and I was sure they'd reached their decision while Sanford was being X-rayed. The wife began to cry while the husband explained to me that they simply couldn't afford to spend that much money on the dog. True, they loved him, but they'd already spent more than they should have. There were lots of free healthy dogs around and, though it would disappoint their children, who had come to think of Sanford as a family member, they'd have to put him to sleep and one day soon get another dog.

As his death sentence was read Sanford sat in his awkward splay-legged puppy position on the steel table panting happily and twitching the end of his tail. Despite my experience, I'm not really made for these situations so, as the wife cried and petted Sanford, my eyes became wet too. I was about to pick him up and take him to a holding cage in the back when the woman put a hand on my arm and stopped me. "Dr. Haddock," she said, "if there's any way you can do the operation anyhow and then give Sanford to another family, that would be wonderful. I can't stand the thought of him dying if he can be helped. He's such a great dog."

By then the husband was getting teary and he took his wife's arm and steered her out of the office. I was left alone with Sanford, but at the prospect of operating on him and finding him another home, I was considerably more cheerful.

Sanford was teetering on the brink between puppyhood and dogdom. The word that would best describe him at that rite of passage was "goofy." He was too big for his body and was always forgetting one of his paws or chewing on his tail or lying down too fast and hitting his head. He soon became a favorite around the hospital. Because the owners had given permission, I was going to perform the surgery on Sanford, but as I'd never done the procedure before I had to wait until someone who had was around to watch me. Several days went by and my schedule never coincided with the right surgeon's schedule and so finally someone else operated on Sanford.

Sanford had recovered nicely. Thin immediately following the operation, he soon began to put on weight and was even beginning to lose some of his goofiness. Perhaps the experience of surgery had affected him because he acquired a look of wisdom that he managed to maintain constantly, except when he chewed on his tail.

This was the Sanford who would be sharing Christmas with me the next day and he filled my thoughts on Christmas Eve. After all, I was responsible for having Sanford at the animal hospital and I would soon have to do something about finding him a home. The hair had grown back over his incision. He was fully recovered and fat and happy and would make someone a wonderful pet. Moreover, for his own good I didn't think it made sense to keep him much longer. A young dog needs a family to socialize him. He needs to get attached to people while he's young so he can become a loving and loyal pet. Sanford had great potential as a family pet but he was soon going to turn into a "kennel dog" if he stayed with us. The sooner Sanford found his family, the better.

I finally fell asleep on Christmas Eve determined to spend Christmas finding a new home for Sanford. I'd go through the hospital files until I found some likely candidates—families who, in my opinion, needed a new dog. Then as soon as possible I'd begin making calls. But on Christmas morning I awoke with a new and even better plan for Sanford's future.

I had to be at work by noontime, but I had a few things to do first. I had decided to take Sanford back home—back to his original home with his original family, who, after all, loved him so much that, with the wisdom of Solomon, they were willing to give him up so he could be happy with another family. It would be the best Christmas present I could give anyone. It certainly would make my lonely Christmas a memorable one. Once I'd made my decision, I had a brainstorm as to how to go about it.

I called one of the few friends I had in Pittsburgh. Jim was from a large Catholic family and, just as I suspected, they were all home on Christmas morning. It sounded like there were thousands of them in the background but Jim assured me that there were only eight or nine. More would be arriving later in the day.

Hearing their muffled voices made my apartment seem deathly quiet and I was reminded of how much I wanted to create a big boisterous family for myself one day. I thought briefly of Dave and how he was no doubt spending Christmas with his large family on their farm. I had dated lots of people since Dave but I hadn't found anyone I'd want to share my life with. Now that I was working, and working peculiar hours, it was difficult to meet men. That morning on the phone with Jim I suddenly felt very alone. Perhaps my dreams of a future that included a family and some version of a white picket fence would *never* be. My work was the driving force in my life and in that moment it struck me as peculiar that though I believed two things were crucial to my happiness— work and family—I could devote my attention to only one while the other would have to occur by luck or by accident.

I told Jim about Sanford and made my proposal concerning Sanford's presentation as the best Christmas gift this side of the Mississippi. Jim was immediately excited about my idea, and he took a quick family conference while I held on. I could tell from the escalation in noise level that they were as enthusiastic as Jim so we made plans to meet in a group in an hour at Castle Shannon.

I drove through the snow and got to the hospital with just

enough time to make a crucial phone call. Flipping through the records, I found Sanford's original file and the phone number of his owners. I dialed the number and when a woman answered I asked if "Susie" was there. The familiar voice said that I must have the wrong number. The first hurdle was crossed; they were at home. I had two more hurdles: I had to find a giant red bow and I had to find out if Sanford's family really wanted him back.

The red bow was easy. After a few minutes of fruitless searching I remembered the giant wreath on the front door. As it was Christmas Day I didn't think anyone would mind if I took the bow. It was being impounded for a worthy cause. I untied the bow and took it to the back room, where Sanford was curled in his cage. His tail began to thump when he saw me. It had been a particularly lonely few days for him. The usual quick pace of the hospital had slowed for the holidays. He'd been having his daily walks of course, but there wasn't nearly as much activity as usual and I think his solitude was weighing on him as much as mine was on me.

The minute I opened his cage door Sanford was out and wagging, goofy as could be in his excitement at this unexpected company. Tying a ribbon on a Labrador retriever who's determined to do nothing but lick your face is wet work, but within a few minutes Sanford was looking very spiffy, some might say even foppish, with his giant bow. The bow was approximately one quarter his size and the contrast between its bright red color and the shiny black of Sanford's coat was classically appealing.

I'd just gotten Sanford's belongings packed—his original collar and leash, his favorite rubber bone—when Jim and his brothers and sisters arrived. As I didn't know Pittsburgh very well, Jim checked the file to see if he knew where Sanford's family lived. It was a stroke of luck that they were just a few blocks from the hospital. It was while Jim was checking the address that I got cold feet. "Jim, do you really think this is a good idea? What if they don't want him? Maybe they already have another dog. What if just the sight of him makes them feel bad?"

"Sally," Jim said, looking incredulous, "are you kidding? Just look at that dog." Sanford had adopted a dignified air and was sitting on the floor holding very still, as if in an effort to be worthy of his bow. "He's fabulous. Who could resist him? Besides"—he nodded toward the waiting room where his family could be heard tuning up for the event—"you're out-numbered. They're so excited about this that I'm afraid it's out of your hands. Believe me"—he grinned—"I know what they're like once they get started." No doubt Jim knew best about the determination of his siblings. And he was right about Sanford: no one could resist him.

We piled into two cars—Sanford got the window without protest from any quarter—and in a very short time we arrived at our destination. Fortunately there was a nice stand of ever-greens a few feet from the front door and Sanford and I took up our positions hidden behind the trees. As the snow fell all around them, Jim and his siblings began to sing Christmas carols. First was "O Come, All Ye Faithful." There were ten people singing and they ranged in age from about five to twenty-three. I knew that Jim's family liked to sing but I'd never heard them before. Now I knew that singing was not only a pleasure for them, it was a family gift. As they har-monized on the "O Come let us adore Him" stanza they sounded like angels.

Midway through the first carol, the curtain parted on the inside door and a woman looked out. When she saw that it was Christmas carolers, she opened the inside door with a big smile. Soon her husband joined her and then, as the window on the storm door steamed up, I could make out one, two and then four little faces pressed to the glass. Despite the snow and the cold, my hands were sweating. This was going to be either wonderful or a major disappointment. Sanford's heart was pounding against mine and those two thumps seemed to me almost as loud as the carols. Finally Jim and company launched into "We Wish You a Merry Christmas." It was my signal. Midway through the short song I left my hiding place with the beribboned Sanford, who was getting too large to hold.

The woman noticed first. I could see the smile leave her face as she recognized my face and then Sanford, who was wiggling in my arms. But what I took for dismay was simply surprise. At the same moment that Sanford realized he was home, the rest of his family recognized him. The storm door swung open. The woman rushed out into the snow. Jim and his family kept singing. The woman was crying and everyone tumbled out the door after her. "Sanford! Is it Sanford?" But they knew it was. He leaped from my arms and threw himself at his family, wagging and grinning, all his dignity lost and his bow slipping until it rested beneath his chin. With moist eyes, Jim and his choir finished their chorus.

It was one of the finest Christmases I can remember, and as I spent the rest of the day taking emergencies and doing routine housekeeping chores back at Castle Shannon, I kept thinking of the moment when everyone, including Sanford, knew that he had come home at last.

HARDWARE DISEASE

After months at Castle Shannon I began to yearn for something more. I remembered my preceptorship at the Animal Medical Center in New York with fondness. The bustling days, the wonderful camaraderie and the endless flow of interesting cases. The AMC offered an internship program for vets and it wasn't long before I decided that was what I wanted. With the encouragement of friends, I applied and then settled back down to work at Castle Shannon. But it wasn't long before my acceptance arrived. I was to be an intern at the AMC. I was almost as excited as I had been when I'd been accepted in vet school. But it was only spring and the internship didn't begin until July.

During that summer the question of the Pennsylvania State Boards came up. In order to practice as a vet in the United States you need to pass the state board exam of the particular state in which you want to work. By the time I finished school I knew that I would be working in Pennsylvania but I hadn't yet taken the Pennsylvania boards. When I graduated I took the national boards and the Ohio State Boards and then, when I knew I'd be working at Castle Shannon, I'd gotten a temporary Pennsylvania license. I figured I'd take the PA boards soon after I was working there. But once it came time to take them, I knew I'd be going to the Animal Medical Center in New York. There seemed little point in bothering with the boards for a state I'd probably never practice in again. When I announced my decision to skip the PA boards to my boss he suggested I take them just for the heck of it. After all, I'd already paid the fee and as it didn't really matter how I did, I could be relaxed about it. Besides, I would now be facing the New York boards, which are supposed to be extremely difficult, so the Pennsylvania boards would give me a painless dry run.

There's nothing like the warm feeling you have the night before a test you don't have to study for. After years of intensive studying, the night before the PA boards was more fun for me than most artificial methods of merrymaking. I relaxed, watched a little television, which I rarely do, and then went out with some friends to have a few beers. I got home just before midnight and, savoring my confidence in the face of a test that I was taking cold, I opened one of my large-animal textbooks. As there are lots of large animals in Pennsylvania, I reasoned, they'd probably be asking lots of questions on them. Large animals have always been my weak point. But who cared? Tomorrow was a free day. Nonetheless I happened to open the book to a disease that I'd forgotten about. Upon seeing the text and photo I recalled laughing about "hardware disease" back in my student days. Hardware disease is a malady that cows get from eating, you guessed it, hardware. As they graze, they pick up nails and bolts and other metal implements that fall off farm machines. Whether cows would eat nails if you gave them a bucketful is a question that bears scrutiny. Anyhow, the cows are well content with eating hardware except for one thing. The nails and other materials land in one of the cow's stomachs and from there can migrate up into the chest cavity where they can puncture the sac surrounding the heart, called the pericardium, which leads to all sorts of serious complications and infections.

The prevention for hardware disease is refreshingly practical, and my guess is credit for its discovery does not belong to sophisticated veterinary research. I can just imagine the scene when hardware disease prevention made its way from folk wisdom to veterinary medicine. The white-coated vet is standing among the only herd of cattle in the area that never gets hardware disease. He's checked out the content of their feed, had their water analyzed and even done mineral tests on the grass and the general nutritional quality of the local dropped hardware. Finally, in total frustration he turns to the farmer and asks what he thinks is a rhetorical question: "I'm stumped. Why are your cows well while every other bovine in the neighborhood has hardware disease?" The farmer shifts his chaw to the other cheek. "Thought you'd never ask, Doc. The trick is, ya feed 'em magnets. Gits 'em polarized and keeps the damn nails under control. Never fails." Another medical breakthrough.

Sure enough, the prevention for hardware disease is magnets. You take your average cow and your magnet and before she ever gets a chance to chomp down on that first bolt you shove a magnet down her throat. She gulps it down and maybe even likes it and asks for more, but there's no need for overkill on magnets. You don't want your herd levitating at full moon. The heavy magnet sits in the cow's stomach and all those bolts and nails and lost screwdrivers and monkey wrenches and bits of farm implements find their way to the magnet where they sit harmlessly. The cow gets heavy and a little low-slung but stays healthy. I suppose after she's lived to the fullness of her years, the farmer can open her up and retrieve a few year's inventory of hardware supplies. It's hard to imagine I could forget hardware disease existed but I had. So that night I went to sleep thinking about giant magnetized cows.

The Pennsylvania State Boards began at nine in the morning and I was there right on time. There were two parts. First we took the written section. For the second year in a row, Pennsylvania was experimenting with latent-image exams. I've mentioned them before because we'd taken them in vet school. They're useful for giving a thorough workout to a student because you can't get away with a simple "true" or "false" or a letter answer. Best of all, as far as the examiners are concerned, they are progressive: if you're supposed to be diagnosing an animal's disease there are a number of things you could do once you know the symptoms. On a latent-image exam, you move through all your choices. If you make a slightly wrong choice you can still continue. If you make a terrible choice, the test announces that you've killed the patient and are facing a malpractice suit. Much like real life.

There were a lot of sheep questions on the PA boards. I struggled through them, hoping for the best, but I confess that by the time I'd finished, I'd been slapped with at least one malpractice suit. The confidence that had propelled me all morning was beginning to wane. Even though it didn't matter, I didn't want to fail. Or, if I failed, I wanted to do it privately. But that might be impossible because I was about to begin the oral boards. Oral tests can be a strain because you're performing as well as thinking. I can manage this dual feat without too much trouble, but due to the death of the sheep on the written exam, my confidence was beginning to ebb, and I was now coping with the embarrassment factor.

When I entered the room there were three examiners—two men and a woman. They did their best to relax me by asking where I'd studied and where I would be practicing. Then the pleasantries were over. The lady examiner went first. She asked me what I'd look for on an X ray of a cat if I suspected it had feline asthma. I answered that without any trouble. The next examiner asked me what kind of a diet I would recommend for a puppy that had suffered a broken leg. Aha! I thought, the trick question. It's too easy. But I dove in. I said I'd give it a normal puppy food along with some extra calcium or maybe some cottage cheese if the dog was especially fussy. It was a score. The only thing that was wrong was my assumption about the trick question; it had really been just a simple, basic one. When the last examiner smiled at me I knew I had it coming. His speciality was large animals — my weakest area. He hunkered down on the table and dropped his little bomb. "Tell me what you know about hardware disease." Hardware disease! What joy! What a sense of triumph! I gave a description of hardware disease that would have impressed even a cow. As I warmed to my subject, the mood in the room changed. This was a girl who knew her stuff. I discussed the syndrome, its effects and prevention. It was so completely fresh in my mind, I could have been reciting from the textbook.

Sure enough, I passed my Pennsylvania boards and I still get grateful feelings when I think about all those cows with magnets in their stomach and all those pastures filled with nails.

AMC INTERNSHIP

THE VERY UPPER EAST SIDE

It was time to move back to "the Big Apple." I'd found an apartment and a part-time job and I'd have just enough time to settle in before I began my internship at the AMC.

This time I would be living alone with only Myriah to keep me company. No roommates, no cats, no sleeping on the kitchen floor. I hadn't seen the apartment and I'd been in New York long enough as a preceptor to have some idea of what I should expect, but still, when I arrived at my new place on Sixty-fifth Street between York and First avenues I was mystified. I knew my apartment would have a tub in the kitchen and for $275 a month I didn't mind the inconvenience. But now that I was actually in the apartment, standing in the center of one of its two rooms, single room, surrounded by my suitcases, I couldn't find the tub. The bathroom had only a commode— no sink, no shower—so there had to be a tub or shower somewhere. I poked into every corner and finally gave up. I plopped down at the makeshift dining table to figure things out, and when I rested my elbows on the table, it shifted. When I examined it more closely, I discovered that the table was hiding my bathtub. The "table" was really a door resting on top of the tub. As I rarely would be dining and bathing simultaneously, this seemed a sensible arrangement.

Now the challenge was to walk around the sofa bed once it was unfolded. The room was simply too small to allow for this, so after many fruitless attempts I developed a new routine. Each night before I went to bed I laid my morning clothes on top of the covers. That way I could dress on the bed or in the kitchen without having to gain access to the closet or my bureau.

I arrived several months before my internship started and was lucky enough to get a part-time job immediately at a practice on the Upper East Side of the city and after my first few days at work I knew I was experiencing a world that I'd never encountered before. I was learning all about rich people and their pets. Now most of the clients at this practice were delightful but, to be honest, some of them were difficult. In all my experience thus far, I always concentrated on the animals—any problems that came up were with them. Perhaps they bit or perhaps they wouldn't take medication or perhaps they simply wouldn't respond to treatment. But now I was finding that there were times when the clients needed special treatment as well. For example there was Mrs. Romano.

Mrs. Romano's husband kept a large portion of the city in tortellini by means of his chain of Italian restaurants. New Yorkers are addicted to good Italian food and they'll go to great lengths to get some. I suppose that having that kind of power over people went to Mrs. Romano's head, and by the time she found her way to us with her miniature white poodle, she was too hot to handle. We couldn't do enough for her.

To begin with, there was some question about whether or not the dog was sick. I was on duty when Mrs. Romano arrived and I had a half-dozen clients waiting. Mrs. Romano didn't have an appointment but she nonetheless demanded to see a vet immediately. Her complaint was that she had just been walking the dog and he had had a bout of diarrhea. I had by then been at this practice long enough to know that some Upper East Side dogs get very peculiar cases of diarrhea indeed. It seems that if you are getting your carpet cleaned or going away for a couple of days or having a special party and your dog or cat is going to be in the way, you simply drop it off at the vet's, complain of diarrhea and get the pet admitted. Then, when the party's over, you stop by and pick up the animal. If you have lots of money, it's worth the few hundred dollars it can cost to get a safe, supervised kennel at the last minute.

I suppose this sort of thing happens everywhere but I found it a dramatic contrast to my preceptorship at the AMC only a few blocks away. There we were treating pets who were often desperately sick. We had clients who would skip a meal so they could get their pet treated. We had elderly people who were frightened to bring their pets to us because of the expense and landed on our doorstep only because they loved their animals so much they didn't want to live without them. Of course we had wealthy clients, too, but somehow the emphasis was always on fast, expert treatment and we simply didn't have time to waste on human foibles.

All these things went through my mind when I was paged with Mrs. Romano's emergency. Nonetheless it *was* possible that the dog was severely sick and needed immediate attention, so when Mrs. Romano arrived I saw her before the waiting appointments. She was an imposing figure, with her jet-black hair and her luxurious white fur coat. In fact, she was holding her poodle to her bosom and the dog matched the color of the coat so exactly that at first, seeing the eyes and the movement of white fur, I thought she had brought the fur in for treatment. But once I'd located the dog I realized that we did in fact have a conventional pet on our hands. As I suspected, the dog was in fine fettle and if he'd had any diarrhea it was probably from eating leftover lasagna. But at Mrs. Romano's insistence I admitted him for observation. I told her to call the next day and I'd let her know how her pet was doing.

The next day was a busy one. Very early that morning we'd spent some time at a popular discotheque, the Red Parrot, clipping the nails on the parrots that called the place home. It had been fun to see the disco, which was being talked about as a "hot spot," and I enjoyed telling my friends that, yes, I'd been to the Red Parrot, as if I were a regular. Of course I always wound up telling the truth, and clipping birds' nails is not nearly as impressive as dancing with celebrities, but still I'd talked to the birds that talked to the stars.

When we returned to the office we were already backed up with clients and in the middle of the afternoon I was paged. Mrs. Romano was there to pick up her dog. Now it takes a few minutes to release an animal. We have to give them a final check to be sure they are perfectly clean, fill out forms and often prescribe medication. I couldn't simply send a kennel aide to return Mrs. Romano's pooch. But I was working at that moment on an animal that needed immediate care and I had a list of people who had made appointments in advance waiting patiently in the reception area. Annoyed, I took a minute to dash into the waiting room and tell Mrs. Romano I was sorry that I couldn't help her right away because I had a list of clients waiting. I told her in what I hoped was a sweet voice that I had asked her to call in advance and if she had I could have gotten all the forms filled out and the dog ready to go. As it was, she would have to wait for a few minutes. Mrs. Romano drew herself to her full if unimpressive height, lifted her chin and, with eyes blazing, told me that she simply *couldn't* wait.

At that moment my fantasy began. I had heard of what is known as "rage behavior" in cats. Cats suffering from this peculiar syndrome act as if they're enraged. They hiss, lunge and attack and they're truly terrifying. Once, when I'd been a preceptor at the AMC, I'd been sent to a client's apartment to pick up a cat suffering from rage behavior. The owner, terrified of his pet's sudden inexplicable violence, locked the cat in a closet and now couldn't get his tuxedo out, which he needed for an important event that night. I had to catch and subdue the cat, rescue his tux and take the cat to the AMC for treatment. The causes of rage behavior are not documented, but at the AMC they theorized that it could be connected to an infection in the reproductive tract as it occurs exclusively in intact females.

As Mrs. Romano stood before me I suddenly saw her not as simply an angry rich woman, but as the first case of rage behavior in humans. I also had a theory that perhaps rage behavior in humans could be connected with the ingestion of too much tomato sauce. It's from just such hunches that medical history is made, and knowing that I could be on the verge of a breakthrough helped me to adopt the detached attitude of a scientist as I dealt with Mrs. Romano. In the best of all possible worlds, I would be able to admit her to the clinic, sedate her and put her in our largest and most comfortable cage for observation. If I cut off her vitello tomato for a few days perhaps I would see some improvement in her behavior.

Mrs. Romano snapped me out of my reverie. "Dr. Haddock, I can't hang around here"—at this point she glanced with a sneer at her fellow pet owners in the waiting room—"all day as you seem to expect. I'm in a hurry."

Well, things were going from bad to worse. Now I had a roomful of people watching to see how I would handle rage behavior. The audience had something at stake because they had all made appointments and were now waiting longer than they should have because of the morning backup. The last thing I wanted was the first case of *infectious* rage behavior in humans so I decided that, short of a tranquilizer gun, I'd have to rely on reason.

"I'm really sorry, Mrs. Romano. I have an animal on the table being treated right now and I shouldn't even have left him to talk to you. We have other critical animals waiting for care. I'm going to have to ask you to be as patient as these other people." I admit I was playing to the crowd with that last remark, but I was beginning to lose my scientific perspective and needed all the support I could find. "It will just be a few more minutes. I hate to make you wait, but as I told you, if you'd call in advance we could see you much more quickly."

Perhaps it was the lumping of Mrs. Romano with the hoi polloi in the waiting room. Perhaps it was simply a symptom of rage behavior, but Mrs. Romano could take no more. With a stern look that made me want to duck, she said with Hollywood-style drama, "You'll be sorry you treated me this way, my dear."

I haven't treated you at all, I thought, but if you'd like me to admit you I'd be happy to. But Mrs. Romano was spinning on her alligators and slamming the door behind her.

I rushed back to the animal I was working on with a brand-new feeling. For the first time in my professional experience I was uncertain about how I had handled a patient. I'd never before had any but the best relations with my clients. But now I was seeing a new situation. Should I have seen her right away? But what about this animal that needed my attention and deserved it? And what about all the other people waiting outside? On the other hand, this wasn't my practice. It was, after all, a business and not mine. Would my boss be angry with me? Had I lost Mrs. Romano for him as a client? What exactly were the ethics of such a situation?

I can't say I came up with any answers but I was preoccupied with the problem all day. I was seeing my job in a new light and I wasn't sure I understood or wanted to understand all the implications.

I spoke with my boss the next day about the Romano encounter and if he was angry with me he didn't let on. Mrs. Romano had called him, eager to fill him in on the rudeness of his "help" and she had told him that she wouldn't be back, that she didn't need to bother with this sort of treatment. I decided not to tell my boss about my theory on rage behavior in humans. Sometimes science has to work slowly and protect itself from unbelievers. But I explained the situation to him. He hated to lose a client but at the same time he had experienced Mrs. Romano himself and so was sympathetic to my course of action.

Weeks passed and Mrs. Romano was forgotten. Until one day months later. I was hard at work one morning in the first month of my internship at the AMC. When "walk-in cases" arrive at the AMC they are assigned to a medical service and one vet on the service is designated as "walk-in" doctor.

This particular morning I was rushing from one case to the next, busy as I ever thought I could be. I'd just finished dealing with a cat with a heart problem—congestive cardiomyopathy. I knew the cat should be put to sleep as its prognosis was very poor, but I also knew that the woman who owned it was having great difficulty making this decision. I was trying to help the cat by giving it medication to stop its pain while I encouraged the woman to face her decision. I find these cases particularly difficult. When I glanced at the chart to see what new cases had been assigned to me I wasn't really paying much attention. Then suddenly I was completely alert. My next patient was a miniature poodle who was in for diarrhea. He was owned by a Mrs. Romano.

Was someone playing a joke on me? But no one at the AMC knew about my encounter with the First Lady of Pasta. Was this a trial sent by God? What would Mrs. Romano say if she saw me calling her into an examining room? Would the inevitable fireworks be worth the expression on her face? Life is a deep well, I thought, recalling the all-purpose axiom I first heard from an inebriated patron discussing foreign policy at the Luv Pub in my waitressing days.

Holding the card with Mrs. Romano's name on it, I convinced a fellow intern to take the case. I did it for the AMC and for Mrs. Romano and for myself. I knew that I could subsist in the city even if I were blacklisted from every Italian restaurant. But I wasn't sure that Mrs. Romano and the AMC would emerge happily from the *mano a mano* confrontation that would surely result if I got involved in treating her dog. Discretion was the better part of valor.

NEW YORK BOARDS

As I waited to begin my internship at the AMC in July, only one cloud loomed on the horizon: the New York State

Boards. In order to practice in New York, I'd have to take them and they were known to be the toughest in the country. Most of the new interns at the AMC would be taking them together in June. They were only given twice a year—in June and December. In what seemed a cruel twist of timing as far as the new interns were concerned, you didn't get your grades until nearly September. By then you were three months into your internship working on the basis of a temporary license, but if you failed the boards you were yanked from the AMC and couldn't come back because your temporary license was rescinded and you couldn't practice in New York until you had a permanent license. Later, when the grades came in, I saw how disappointing it was for interns to have to leave their jobs and, in effect, postpone their lives for a year in the hope they'd pass the next time around.

Because I was working at the Upper East Side practice part-time that spring in New York, I had more flexibility than most. So I took advantage of my situation and flew up to Ithaca, New York, two weeks before the boards were given to have my own private study session. Cornell University, in Ithaca, is the site of the New York State Boards and students from all over the country and the world were there studying when I arrived. It must have driven the regular Cornell students batty because every year they were driven out of their library and robbed of their facilities so the great influx of vet students could cram for the boards. Foreign vet students—ones who have studied outside the United States—are particularly frenzied because most of them have never had access to facilities similar to those at Cornell. They are usually far behind American students clinically as they have had very little exposure to clinics. Desperate to catch up, many of them come to Cornell six months before the test to study.

I was at Cornell for five days but I was so busy the whole time that it seemed like weeks. My major fear was the large-animal portion of the exam. In the Cornell library they had books of large-animal breeds. I spent hours with those books as well as with flash cards of cows and pigs and sheep, trying to memorize every variation. They also had slide carousels filled with slides of large-animal breeds and after a day of books and slides and flash cards I began to see large animals everywhere.

It's not too difficult to distinguish between pig breeds. Red pigs, should you ever encounter one, are Durocs; pink pigs with straight ears are Yorkshires. Nubian goats have floppy ears while La Mancha goats have none. Even cows are fairly amenable to being memorized: Holsteins are black and white dairy cows, Jerseys are pretty light-brown cows with long eyelashes. But sheep, for all their benign appeal, are killers when it comes to telling them apart. Perhaps it's the one revenge of an animal with no natural defenses. The differences between the breeds are subtle and difficult to remember. Of course there are the easy ones: Suffolks have black faces and black ears. But others are distinguished, for example, by a bald nose, a half-furred nose, a fully furred nose. So you can have three white sheep who all look alike except for the amount of hair on their noses and even their mothers probably have to look twice to find the right lamb.

While I was trying to get my porcines and bovines in order I was also spending a lot of time in the poisonous plant garden. Cornell has a garden of several hundred poisonous plants and we had to become experts on all of them. We had to be able to identify them and know what systems of the body they affect. We had to know if they caused neurological signs or gastrointestinal signs. We also had to know how to treat any animal who'd eaten them.

Two weeks after I finished my review session at Cornell I went to Philadelphia for more of the same. Every year the AMC sponsors a study session for the New York boards for their new interns. It was an opportunity to meet for the first time the other interns you'd be working with at the AMC. We were all assigned roommates and we trooped into the Red Fox Inn for a two-day review program. After an early breakfast

we began our work day at 9 A.M. with lectures, slide shows
and more poisonous plants. Then after a few hours of theoretical, we'd break into groups for practical work. We studied
bovine diseases, porcine diseases and diseases of goats. We
tested horses for lameness. We did mastitis milk tests on cows
and scrubbed up cattle. By 7 P.M. we were finished and we
went off to party. By the end of the two-day review we had
all learned a great deal—enough we hoped to get us through
the test—and we had become friends.

The last journey in the quest for a New York State license
was the long drive from Philly to Ithaca. We all drove up
together directly from our review session with the hope that
everything we'd learned would lodge firmly in our minds.
There was so much material—what amounted to the extracts
of hundreds of books—that we could believe that every lump
in Route 95, every short stop at a rest area could jar some
microsynapse in our brains and lose some significant bit of
detail.

When we arrived at Ithaca we were treated like criminals.
Which is to say we were photographed and our identification
papers were scrupulously examined. This is to ensure that you
don't send your boss at the clinic or your father the vet up to
take the test for you. It was with a strange mixture of emotions
that I learned the crucial admittance form that had been mailed
to all test takers had never found its way to me. Finally the
powers that be saved me from six more months of anxiety by
at last believing that I was who I said I was.

Most of us had been hearing about the N.Y. boards for
years. The foreign students among us had heard of them from
as far away as Milan or Munich. They had been gossiped
about and dreaded by the assembled crowd for so long that
we all felt we knew everything possible about them except the
answers. The details of the marking system were most important and most ominous: if you failed one out of the four
parts, you could get a temporary license and practice for six
months, when you'd have to take the test again; if you failed

two parts or more you couldn't practice in New York until you passed the next time around. We were all aware of what the schedule of the particular tests would be. On the first day we'd be doing equine and small animals. On the second day we'd do bovine and miscellaneous. Miscellaneous covers poultry, swine and laboratory animals.

As far as I was concerned, this was a fine schedule. I felt confident about small animals and fairly confident about horses. I should be able to move through them confidently the first day. Then, bovine, which had always given me the most trouble, was on the second day and I'd have some extra time to study it.

On the morning of the first day we were broken into two groups. Half of us would be taking the first set of tests while the other half of us would take the other. In the afternoon we would switch subjects. "So," said the announcer, "we'll have the bovine people exit through this door and the small-animal people exit through this one." The cry went up instantly: "*Bovine?* It's supposed to be horses." But it was too late. Somewhere the mistake had already been made. Those who had spent the night studying horses were out of luck. And those who were weak in bovine were in trouble. Great, I thought, I'm doing poorly before I even begin. But someone was watching out for me: I was in the group that was destined to take small animal first. At least I'd have lunchtime to study bovine.

We gathered in one room and began to wait our turn for the small-animal exam. Finally they called my number and I soon was standing before a table that held an anesthetized cat. The cat had an arrhythmia of the heart, which is one of the side effects of a blocked cat. They wanted to know what type of arrhythmia it was. At the next station we were given needles and instruments and asked to do various sutures. This was home turf to me and I felt at ease. But when I got to the next station my confidence wavered. There was a dog who was suffering from nicotine poisoning and they wanted to know what symptoms to look for and how to treat it.

Though I was up to date on my poisonings, nicotine was one I wasn't sure of. In fact, I couldn't recall ever having heard of it as an animal poison. Had this dog taken up smoking? Oh why couldn't this dog have eaten some warfarin, the rat poison I know so well? As a preceptor at the AMC I'd spent lots of time working with warfarin poisonings. Warfarin is a common rat poison that the city puts out at various times of the year to keep the rat population from taking over Gracie Mansion. Lots of it goes into Central Park and occasionally dogs who use the park eat it and get very sick. It's a potentially deadly poison if it goes untreated and many pets who eat it die. Warfarin interferes with the clotting system and the antidote is vitamin K[1] and in severe cases blood transfusions are required. Some vets and even people know that you treat warfarin with vitamin K but they don't use vitamin K[1] and therefore are not successful. At any rate, I was very familiar with that and any and every plant poison after all my time in the Wicked Witch gardens. But nicotine I wasn't sure of.

I answered the questions as well as I could, keeping my fingers crossed. But I was feeling a little shaky. I had seven more stations to go and from that poor poisoned dog it all seemed downhill. There was one question after another that I wasn't sure of.

When I came out of the small-animal exam I was devastated. I had taken one part, my speciality, and I felt like I'd blown it. I could feel myself beginning to go into a downward spiral, reaching that point when the spirit won't cooperate and the will is gone and blunder can be the only result. If I were a horse, they would have taken me out and shot me. Realizing that, I knew that I'd have to pull myself together and do the best I could. Heads up, heads up, I kept saying to myself as I went into the bovine exam.

At the very beginning of the tests you are given a number and you're known throughout the two days by that number. This is to keep any political questions about passing certain people and failing others at bay. No one who is examining you is supposed to know who you are or where you came from. But the Cornell vet students wear green coveralls and the general feeling is that, if anything, the examiners will lean in favor of a native son. With this in mind, many of the students, particularly the foreigners, had gone out and bought green coveralls. I couldn't see doing this and so there I was, one of the few blues or whites in a sea of green. My blue coveralls became significant at the end of the bovine exam.

Much to my surprise I felt that I was doing well throughout the bovine section. All the material was fresh in my mind. In fact, my feeling of success made me think that as far as my study time was concerned, I had neglected small animal in favor of bovine. Finally I came to the last station of the first part of the bovine. I felt the examiner looking hard at my blue coveralls. Then came the last question: every state in the U.S. has a number for tagging cattle so they can be traced back to the state of origin. What was the number for New York State. I understood why he had been staring at my blue coveralls. As it was clear I wasn't from Cornell and therefore not from New York State, it was highly unlikely I would know the New York State number. He had a sympathetic look in his eyes as he waited for my answer. I hesitated, grinned and said, "Well, obviously my blue coveralls are a giveaway. I'll have to make a guess." Of course it had to be from one to fifty and I knew Ohio's number so that meant I had forty-nine guesses. "Twenty-one?" I said. His jaw dropped. The examiners weren't supposed to tell us how we'd done on a question but it was obvious by his expression that New York's number was twenty-one. Breaking the rules, he smiled and said, "*Aw-right!*"

After that there was no stopping me. I still had a few more sections of bovine to go but I was feeling good. Finally I came to the last question, which was set up like a combination fun-house/peep-show attraction. Before you was a white board with three holes in it. On the other side of the board were three bovine reproductive systems. You picked your number, put on your glove and reached in to examine the system of your choice. I had to determine if my mystery cow was pregnant. Well, I reached in and this cow was so pregnant that if I'd waited a few minutes I'd have been able to pull out a calf. "Pregnant," I said with a smile.

By the end of the first day I felt there was a good chance that I'd failed the small animal but also certain that I'd done well on bovine. That meant I had to pass both miscellaneous and equine the next day if I wanted to keep my temporary license. That night I studied over dinner and a few beers with a Cornell student. I was one of the few Ohio students to be so relaxed: the others were hardly taking time to eat. But I figured that there was no great advantage to frenzied preparation at this late stage.

The next morning, horses were first. We had to face a horse and as the examiner named various parts we had to point to where they were located on the animal. Then he would name various diseases and we'd have to indicate the affected part of the horse's body. It was difficult but I thought I'd done fine. Then we had to look at various X rays of joints and legs of horses that had something wrong with them and tell what the X ray revealed and give the prognosis. Then we had to describe how to treat the problem. Then, at last, I got to use my poisonous plant knowledge in a section that asked us to identify plants. We also had to identify a series of drugs and name the correct dosages. That was a tough series. Still I felt if luck was on my side, I had passed.

Now I had to face miscellaneous. Everyone had flunked this section the previous year. Moreover, I knew I'd *have* to pass it because I'd most likely flunked small animal. So I entered the miscellaneous room with trepidation. First there were swine parts that had lesions like diamond-skin disease, for example, and you had to identify the disease on the evidence of the lesion. After a few more sections we came to the *very* miscellaneous part of the exam. We were asked to select a lab animal. There was a hamster or a rabbit. With fond memories of Watson, who had eaten all of Skid's plants back in school, I picked a rabbit. Then I had to describe what its diet would be. Then I was asked how I'd restrain the rabbit. The important thing to remember about handling rabbits is that their backs can be easily broken. You have to hold the scruff of their neck with one hand and cradle their back legs with another. As I'd spent so much time with Watson I was a pro. Finally I had to name three common diseases and I rattled them off with no trouble: coccidia, snuffles, ear mites. At last it was chicken time and I breezed through the birds handily. It was over. I was finished. But my prognosis was mixed. I certainly passed bovine, I thought I passed equine and miscellaneous, I probably failed small animal.

Three months later I was working at the AMC and we all knew that the board scores had come in. Over the PA system, one by one, each of the interns was being told to call a certain number. The head of medicine of the AMC gets the scores even before we do and he was calling us in with the news. There was an electricity in the air, that mix of revulsion, fear, excitement that overtakes people watching automobile accidents and people waiting to learn their New York State Veterinary Board scores. At last my name was called. I passed. I passed all four sections, including small animals.

I celebrated when I graduated from Miami U. and when I graduated from Ohio State Vet School. I also celebrated when I got into the AMC as a preceptor and as an intern. But those pale when compared to the celebration when I passed my New York boards. It seemed like a whole part of my life was over.

HIGH-RISE CATS

From the very beginning of my internship at the AMC I loved it. There were no doubts or hesitations about whether or not I'd done the right thing to leave a practice and, in effect, go back to school. I loved the intensity, the camaraderie and the extraordinary range of cases I saw. Because the AMC is at the forefront of animal medicine they see difficult cases regularly that get referred to them for treatment and consultation. Each was an education in itself. But there was another kind of education available with the regular day-to-day clinic cases. As I had in North Carolina, New Hampshire and Pennsylvania, I began to see common syndromes that were peculiar to New York City.

The fact that geography is a determining factor for vets as far as what they regularly treat holds as true for Manhattan as the wilds of western Pennsylvania or the woods of New Hampshire. It seems strange to use the word "geography" in relation to New York City. "Geography" always means to me mountains, rivers, plateaus, wetlands and rolling plains. Nothing, save perhaps Central Park, gives any hint of New York geography.

Nonetheless the canyons of New York provide some of their own peculiar cases and I quickly filed away my expertise on fishhooks and moved on to high-rise cats.

High-rise cats are a phenomenon unique to cities where buildings are as tall as engineering permits. In vet circles a high-rise cat is one who makes an unplanned leap from a high floor of an apartment building. Like forsythia and azaleas, they're among the first signs of spring in New York, as people open their windows for the first welcome balmy days after a grim winter.

Many people think that cats, with all their dignity and wisdom, are unaffected by an open window. Cats are smart enough to tell the difference between glass and no glass, they maintain. Or they believe that cats have a sublime sense of balance that permits them to rest on their window ledges safely while napping in the sunshine.

I hasten to inform all cat owners that some cats have a very poor sense of balance. One minute they're humming "Summertime," the next they're tumbling through the air. If you own a cat, you know it's curious. A passing butterfly or bumblebee or pigeon can easily lure it into a dangerous free-fall.

Observations of many cases of high-rise cats have yielded a "floor prognosis." It has been said that the kitties who leap from floors four through seven usually have the worst of it. Falling from a lower floor is, obviously, safer. Falling from a higher one gives the cat a chance to right itself and land on its feet. Of course, as you might imagine, landing on your feet after a fall from the fifteenth story does not mean you've beat the devil; broken paws, shock, a split palate or air in the chest cavity are just a few of the common problems encountered by high-rise cats.

Some high-rise cats survive falls from great heights. One legendary cat fell twenty stories and survived. Canopies and hedges often save a cat's life as they break an otherwise fatal fall. Concrete, however, is unforgiving. I recently had an eleven-month-old cat that had fractured its back in a fall to the concrete sidewalk. It had been found in the bushes and, when I examined it, it had no "deep pain," which means no sensation in its hind legs. This indicates a spinal cord injury and the cat had to be put to sleep. Nothing could be done for it. The owners, new to the city and never guessing their cat could lose its balance, left arm in arm and in tears. It's terrible to know you could have prevented the death of your pet.

Of course no one can save a cat from street crime once it lands on the pavements of New York. The Animal Medical Center was abuzz one spring day with the news of a charming cat that had fallen from a third-story window. Luckily she had landed safely on a patch of grass in front of the building. But she was in heat. While she stood near the doorway of her apartment building dazedly waiting to be rescued, a passing tom cat had his way with her. The streets just aren't safe anymore. And the New York male is an especially perilous breed of cat.

Puffy was one of my most memorable high-rise cats. When Puffy arrived at the Animal Medical Center she was a little

wobbly but in good spirits. The young man who'd brought
her in was, by contrast, frantic. Puffy was in his care until
his fiancée made her long-anticipated move from Baltimore to
New York. Puffy was her cat, and in a few days she'd be in
New York. If all went well in the Big Apple he, the fiancée
and Puffy would eventually be joined in legalized bliss.

Puffy had foiled things by leaping out of a third-story window. Our hero, no great cat enthusiast, had been bustling
about the apartment, cleaning and dusting, and enjoying a
series of beers, when Puffy made her leap. It took a few
minutes before she was missed. Perhaps "missed" is too sen-
timental a word in this case. In any event, eventually our hero
noticed that there was no white cat sitting on his navy-blue
sweater, no kitty munching on his begonia. After a halfhearted
search that included the oven and the laundry hamper, our
hero noticed the open window. On a whimsical and perhaps
hopeful hunch, he leaned out. Puffy was surfing the waves of
the ragged privet hedge that surrounded the building three
stories below. Can this marriage be saved?

When Puffy landed on my examining table she was far
calmer than her keeper. But of course Puffy hadn't had a single
beer. What was he going to *tell* his fiancée? Two weeks with
the cat and he'd driven it to suicide! What kind of a future
did this portend? Where could he get another beer?

Meanwhile, I was examining Puffy. I pressed my stethoscope to her chest. I palpated her abdomen to check for a
ruptured bladder, an occasional result of a fall. I pried open
her mouth and examined her palate. Often when cats manage
to land on their feet, the force of the fall smacks their heads
against the pavement and splits their palates. Finally I gently
massaged her paws in my hands. If they sound like the noise
that made Rice Krispies famous—snap, crackle, pop—the
paws have been broken.

Puffy seemed to be fine. The hedge must have broken her
fall. Nonetheless I decided to X-ray her chest to be sure there
was no free air in her chest cavity. I sent her owner back to

the waiting area while Puffy headed for X ray.

While Puffy's films were being developed her owner was amusing everyone in the waiting room with his tales of premarital guilt and his seeming inability to contend with a small white cat. "If Puffy doesn't pull through," he said melodramatically, "I might lose the woman I love." Puffy the highrise cat had become a symbol of true love, Manhattan style.

When Puffy's X rays were clipped to the light box, I was pleased to determine that her ribs were all intact and there was no air in the chest. But I did see something unusual. I called her caretaker in for a look.

"Is it fatal?" He was wringing his hands. "Please don't tell me I'm a kitty killer. Save me from the singles bar scene! Let Puffy live! How much does all this cost?"

I pointed to the X ray. "There's something that might help when the bill comes."

When our hero pried his fingers from his eyes he saw the faint outlines of George Washington's face in Puffy's midsection.

"This is a joke," he said, his eyes wide. "You doctored the prints. Tell me this is a joke."

A small crowd of vets had gathered. "What you see is what you get," I explained. "Puffy has swallowed a nickel." Someone produced a nickel and fit it precisely over the spot on Puffy's X ray. If you looked closely you could see the shadow of a face and a firm jawline. "Heads," I said.

"She's a thief. First she steals my money, then she tries to make her escape out an open window. That's gratitude for you. I sacrifice my time, my peace and my dark clothes and what do I get? A cat burglar."

The treatment for Puffy's nickel was simple but unappealing, especially in the atmosphere of mistrust that Puffy's theft had created. Our hero had to carefully sift Puffy's litter for a few days to see if the nickel had passed through her system. The coin was in her stomach and it could either pass harmlessly through her intestines, which was unlikely, or it could, at any time, become lodged at the beginning of the intestines. If that happened, Puffy would have to be operated on to remove the nickel.

The prospect of sifting litter was the final indignity. As Puffy was carried through the waiting room I heard our hero offer her to any taker. "Free kitty," he said, holding Puffy aloft, "and a nickel rebate."

LEISHMANIA

As my internship at the AMC continued I handled more and more exotic cases. I spent two weeks working with a vet on Long Island, Dr. Altman, who is a recognized U.S. authority on birds, and I learned a great deal from him. Exotics really interested me, but because of them I was often overloaded on my cases. When exotics came in they were usually sent to me, as the other vets would refuse to see them, and when they were piling on top of my regular load, things would get hectic. Not only did the exotics add to my regular work load, they also generally take more time to treat than a dog or a cat because most of the procedures and medications have to be worked out on a case-by-case basis. For example, getting blood from a hamster can be a challenge. Figuring out how much of an antibiotic to give a parakeet who might weigh thirty grams takes a few minutes to puzzle out.

I had been seeing a lot of lead poisoning in birds. Most often the bird is brought in because it's been having seizures. Lead poisoning is the most common cause of seizures in birds so the first thing I do is get a good history. I have to know if the bird is ever let out of its cage where it might come in contact with a source of lead. In New York the paint on the walls of old apartments is often lead-based. I've seen birds who got lead poisoning from the metal solder that holds Tiffany-style lamps together. They can also get it from eating batteries or linoleum or even from the metal wires around the cork on champagne bottles.

I was just finishing up with my latest case of lead poisoning. A woman had a blue and gold macaw who had suffered repeated seizures. She had taken him to a local vet who had observed him for a few days. The bird was fine for a day or two and then began to have more seizures. Despite the vet's recommendation to put the bird to sleep, the woman refused and desperately sought an alternative. She was attached to the bird and had paid nearly $1,000 for him. Finally she arrived at the AMC for a second opinion.

I examined the bird and took the history and suspected lead poisoning. To detect lead poisoning one takes an X ray and examines it for metallic densities. On an X ray, air appears black and bones are white. But metallic densities are bright, bright white. If a bird, or a dog or a rabbit for that matter, has lead poisoning, you can often see bright metallic densities in the belly. The problem with the X-ray method of detection is that a bird's digestion is so fast the lead chips may pass through the system very quickly and sometimes won't show up on the X ray even though some lead has been absorbed into the bloodstream.

When I saw the macaw's film, I knew he was a case of lead poisoning. His stomach was filled with bright white pellets. The treatment for lead poisoning is injections of calcium EDTA for four to five days. The calcium binds up with the lead in the bloodstream and the animals eventually excrete it. Birds usually need to stay in the hospital for the injections and longer if they have vomiting or diarrhea as a symptom in addition to the seizures. If they're not eating they have to be tube-fed or given fluid injections because they can die very quickly of malnutrition. Their metabolic rates are so rapid that one day of a parakeet not eating is comparable to twenty-five days of a human fast. When you treat a bird for any disease, you have to pay a great deal of attention to supporting the bird as well as curing it: you can cure the disease but, if you're not careful, the bird can quickly die of malnutrition.

I gave the woman with the macaw my diagnosis. How had the bird been poisoned? There was no lead paint in her house and she couldn't think of any other sources of lead the bird had access to. She said the bird chewed on his cage a lot but that shouldn't be the cause of the poisoning because cage manufacturers have strict regulations forbidding the use of lead.

Within several days the bird was doing well enough to go home. I called the owner and told her she could come and get him. In the meantime, she'd solved the mystery. It seems that an analysis for mineral content had proven that there was lead in the bars of the bird's cage. When the woman picked up her macaw she also picked up a copy of his X ray and of our medical reports because she was planning to sue the cage manufacturer, and she certainly had an excellent case.

I was collecting the materials for the macaw owner thinking how I'd welcome a simple case of worms or a cut paw. As a vet you lust for the strange and unusual. Much of the excitement of my work lies in the challenging cases, the mysterious symptoms, the unexpected diagnoses. But with all the exotics and the complicated cases I'd been treating lately, I thought a few days vacation from challenge would be just fine. Well, of course, that's when one of my most challenging cases arrived.

Millie was a black standard poodle. She was two years old and in perfect health except for one thing: she was bleeding from the nose. She was owned by a young Manhattan couple with two children and she was a beloved member of the household. The family had taken her to another vet but he'd been unable to put his finger on the problem so now they were bringing her to the AMC for a second opinion.

In a case like this it's particularly important to get a thorough history of the pet's health. Sometimes, if you don't, you later discover an obvious solution to a seemingly difficult problem and if you'd had a full history you could have saved everyone time and money. So I took Millie's history. She had been hit by a car in February of that year and immediately after the accident she began to bleed from her left nostril. The vet X-rayed her and discovered a hairline fracture in her nose and it was assumed the bleeding was caused by that. Sure enough, the bleeding stopped. Two months later Millie was accidentally kicked in the nose by the little girl and once again her left nostril began to bleed. It seemed obvious the bleeding was caused by the kick and the vet prescribed a tranquilizer to lower Millie's blood pressure and help stop the bleeding. Soon thereafter, the bleeding stopped. A few months later Millie began to bleed occasionally from her nose but this time from both nostrils. This is important because normally a tumor will cause bleeding only on one side unless it's deeply invasive. The vet was at a loss with this third bout of bleeding and he recommended the family take Millie to the AMC.

Once I had her medical history, I got the details of her travel history. With well-traveled dogs you have to consider various parasites that might occur in places the dog has visited. As it turned out, Millie *was* an international dog. She had been born in Virginia but had spent most of her life in Portugal. The family had moved there when Millie was six months old and had lived there until only recently when they'd returned to the United States.

After taking all this information I told Millie's family how I thought best to proceed. I wanted to admit her and do a work-up on her. I figured I'd need a coagulogram to check her clotting factors and platelets to see if there was a clotting problem that could be causing Millie to bleed. If that was normal I'd do skull X rays to see if there was a fracture or a foreign body or a tumor. A tumor could cause the bleeding but you don't expect to find one in a dog so young. When it became clear that Millie would have to spend some time in the hospital, the little girl's eyes became huge and, saying nothing, she looked at her mother, obviously frightened. Seeing her reaction, I spent some time assuring both mother and child that Millie would be fine, that she'd be under constant care and that, if possible, I'd even sneak her a few treats. This seemed to cheer up the child but still she cried when she left the examining room. I was determined to discover the cause of Millie's bleeding.

That afternoon I began the tests. When I checked the referral skull X rays from the original vet, I couldn't see any evidence of a fracture but I decided I'd turn it over to one of our orthopedic specialists. The next morning I got the coagulogram back. There are several things you check in the coagulogram: two tests for clotting factors and the platelet count. If the clotting factors had been off, I would have immediately suspected warfarin, the rat poison, which can cause nosebleeds or bleeding anywhere. But Millie's clotting factors were fine and her platelet count was low.

When I got the coagulogram back and saw the results, I realized Millie was going to be a bit of a puzzle. I mentally checked off the things that could cause low platelets and there was no obvious answer. Millie could have an autoimmune disease called ITP that was causing her body to fight her own platelets. If that were the case we could treat her with steroids and she'd probably live a full life. But I'd have to do further testing to confirm the autoimmune disease. There was also the possibility that Millie had caught a tiny parasite that is usually found in the south or in Puerto Rico called *ehrlicha canis*. But ehrlichiosis affects all the blood cells—red, white and the platelets—and Millie's red and white blood-cell counts were fine. On the other hand, given the dog's travel history, I thought that it was possible for it to be an early stage of ehrlichiosis that hadn't yet affected the red and white cells.

The most common cause of nosebleeds in older dogs is cancer. But Millie had something different. At this point she didn't fit the norm of any disease. It wasn't long before everyone at the AMC knew about her. As I ordered more tests, to check on the autoimmune disease and to check on her bone marrow to see if it was producing platelets that were being destroyed or if it simply wasn't producing any in the first place, Millie became the subject of scrutiny and speculation among the AMC staff.

When the bone marrow test came back, the first pathologist thought he saw evidence of ehrlichiosis but, as we rarely see ehrlichiosis, he wanted a second opinion.

That afternoon, the day after Millie had been admitted to the AMC, I was at a baby shower for a fellow resident. It was my day off but I didn't want to miss this party. As we all stood around chatting, one of the head staff members came up to me and said, "I heard about your dog." "You must mean Millie," I said. "It seems she might have ehrlichiosis." "Worse than that," he replied. "I just heard it might be leishmania."

This information traveled through the crowd like electricity. Leishmania is an extremely rare disease in this country that's spread by sand flies. The shock effect of the leishmania announcement at the party was due only in part to the rarity of the disease; we all well realized that the disease is contagious to humans through a vector. A vector is a crucial element in spreading certain diseases. For example, heartworm in dogs and cats is spread through a vector: the mosquito. An infected dog can't give it to another dog. But if a mosquito—the vector— bites an infected dog, it can then bite an uninfected dog and spread the disease. Sand flies are the vector for leishmania. Millie had no doubt been infected by a Portuguese sand fly. Now if a sand fly bit Millie and then bit a human, the human could get leishmania. As far as we knew there were no sand flies of the particular kind needed to be a vector for leishmania, but could some indigenous insect serve the same function? In any case, as leishmania, if untreated, is a fatal ailment and one that can become epidemic, it was considered a "reportable" disease: we had to report Millie and her leishmania to the federal government.

Once I realized the seriousness of the situation, my mind reeled. There were so many things to consider. Was Millie treatable? Could she infect other dogs? Worse yet, could she infect humans? Were Millie's owners at risk or could they be? And finally, where could I get more information on her disease? The head of medicine at the AMC told me there was a vet in Florida who had recently had a case of leishmania. I called him to learn about his experience. The Florida vet had kept the leishmania dog in contact with some biting flies from

Texas to see if those flies could become a vector and it looked as if they could. The implication was we were now dealing with the possibility of an epidemic: the leishmania potentially could spread without the Portuguese sand flies. Right after I spoke with the Florida vet I learned there had been an extremely rare outbreak of leishmania in Oklahoma which authorities believed had been spread via ticks. Then someone suggested that leishmania could be spread by cockroaches. If that were the case, given the cockroaches in New York and, unfortunately, at the AMC as well, we could be facing a public health emergency. We were all very anxious about Millie and, with this latest news, about ourselves.

I still needed to know if I could begin to treat Millie and so I made a number of calls to find out if that were even possible. First I discovered that cockroaches are not a vector for leishmania, which was an enormous relief. Then I learned that leishmania is treated by administering a heavy metal called antimony. To procure antimony you must report the disease to the state or federal veterinarian and they will be allotted a single dose which they will pass on to you.

By that time we knew a lot about leishmania but we still didn't know for sure if Millie had it. At last we found an expert who could tell us. The second pathologist who examined the results of Millie's bone marrow knew of a woman who was a leishmania expert who was affiliated with New York Hospital. We sent her the slide and waited for word. I couldn't help but reflect on the good fortune both Millie and I had to be at the AMC, where the best medical minds and facilities were available to us.

Meanwhile, as we were testing and consulting, I had explained the situation to Millie's owners. I told them Millie could have ehrlichiosis or she could have leishmania. If it were ehrlichiosis, we could treat it and Millie should do fine. But if it were leishmania, we would have to consider the public health hazard. I could hear the little girl's voice in the background as I spoke. At the sound, Millie was no longer an interesting and challenging case: she was someone's pet. It's a peculiar thing how vets react to disease: if it's something strange and challenging, indeed the sort of thing most likely to worry an owner, it's exciting. However, there are two kinds of excitement: it's most exciting to find that an animal has a strange disease that you can cure. It's exciting to find any other kind of disease, but upon the realization that you can't help the animal, the excitement becomes academic. There's nothing to satisfy but your curiosity. I crossed my fingers and hoped that word from New York Hospital would be encouraging.

That afternoon the family came in to the AMC to visit Millie. They had been missing her and were eager to say hello. Of course the little girl was with them and my heart ached when I saw the red circles around the child's eyes. She must have spent the better part of the past three days crying. The minute she saw Millie, her eyes lit up and she rushed to hug the dog, who was wiggling in ecstasy. I was watching that fond visit when I was paged and I somehow knew that it would be word on Millie. I answered the page and the woman from New York Hospital was on the phone.

"It's leishmania, all right. The first case I ever saw in New York."

I slowly returned to the small examining room where Millie was enjoying her reunion with her family. The mother knew by the look on my face that I had news and it must have been obvious that things looked bleak. I told them that the diagnosis of leishmania had been confirmed. Now the woman's eyes filled with tears. "Can't we take her home? We've been living with her this long and I'm sure we're okay and she'd be much happier at home. And can't you use that metal to treat her?"

I took a deep breath and tried not to look at the little girl. "I'm afraid the prognosis for Millie isn't good. A dog's red blood-cell count is normally thirty-five. When she came in her count was thirty but, with all the bleeding from her nostrils, just in the time she's been here it's gone down to ten. We've been giving her blood transfusions and you couldn't do that at home. Since the leishmania is throughout her bone marrow, the chances of treating it are virtually nil." I was stroking Millie now. "And there's the question of the public health hazard. . . ."

The family was clearly unsure of what to do. They wanted to make the right decision for Millie's sake but they didn't want to cave in to pressure from an establishment that was simply interested in eliminating a problem. All of this I could see on their faces. Then they asked me the question that people so often ask. Usually I'm grateful for them asking it because it allows me to tell them exactly what I think is best. I always answer it honestly. "Dr. Haddock," the mother said, "what would you do if Millie were your dog?"

I thought of Myriah. I watched Millie, wagging her tail as the little girl, eyes still red, held her dog close with one arm while she rubbed her belly. What would I do if it were Myriah? Tears came to my eyes. "I think I'd have her put to sleep."

The family couldn't help but notice my tears and somehow the dynamic of the situation was reversed. The little girl reached over to pat my hand. It was a strange scene in the examining room: four miserable, wet-eyed people and one happy, tail-wagging dog.

The inevitable decision was made. Millie's owners wanted to know if they could take her home and bury her and I had to explain that because the disease was a public health hazard, they couldn't. She would have to be cremated. Now we were all talking through our tears. One instant we'd be smiling self-consciously; the next we'd be blinking furiously, trying to stay in control.

So finally Millie was put to sleep; the little girl went home without her best friend. Eventually the whole family was tested for leishmania but fortunately nothing was found. And one of my most challenging cases became, in retrospect, one of my saddest.

SUE THE GREAT

Though I found my professional life at the AMC exhilarating, my personal life was less than fulfilling. I had plenty of friends and a constant round of activities but I was beginning to wonder if I'd ever meet a man I could take seriously as a potential lifelong partner. The long and complicated hours of veterinary medicine were difficult enough. I was also finding that many of the eligible men I was meeting in New York were mainly interested in casual good times. Or, if they were interested in something more, they were simply not my type. There was a peculiar feeling of being on the wrong side of a supply and demand situation. Even though I dated frequently and met many nice men, I often felt, halfway into an evening, that I was wasting two people's time.

It was May in New York and I was giddy with spring fever. After a blustery and changeable March, at last the weather had become reliably balmy and the tender leaves were bursting from all the trees that had spent the winter scrawny and stick-like against the gray days. I was careening down the ramp into the lobby of the AMC on my way to pick up an order of Chinese food when I was stopped dead in my tracks by a group chatting by the reception desk. There was Steve Birchard, a staff surgeon, two other guys who worked at the AMC and a stranger. It was the sight of the stranger that arrested me. He was tall, with thick sandy hair, blue eyes and a smile that was as refreshingly warm as the spring evening. I edged my way into the conversation and was finally introduced to the mystery man, who turned out to be Steve's brother Tom. After a few minutes I had to excuse myself—people were waiting for their noodles in hot sesame sauce—but I couldn't forget that smile.

At the AMC the staff has what's known as "phone hours." Each of us is assigned a specific half hour during which we take calls from owners whose pets we've treated. We answer questions and update them on their pets' conditions. The phone room has all the charm of a phone booth. It's like a narrow corridor with four phones on each of the two long walls. There is a row of no-nonsense wooden chairs and each time I had phone duty I felt like a prisoner dealing with the outside world. But the aesthetics of the phone room become irrelevant the minute you take your first call and you're swept into the care and concern your clients have for their pets. It's a busy half hour too: usually as you talk to one client, two or three others are on hold waiting for news and information.

It was in the phone room that I next ran into Steve Birchard. I had a rare pause between calls and I passed him a note that said, "Wow, your brother is cute!" Steve turned slowly and dramatically in his chair. Perhaps, I thought, waiting for his reaction, his brother is as married as he is cute. Finally, Steve faced me and, grinning, gave me a memorable if not eluci-dating wink.

A few days later Steve passed me in the hall and when we stopped to chat he invited me to join him and a group of AMC people for an informal dinner later that night. I declined. I had had a long day and was absolutely exhausted. "You must come, Sally," Steve said. "Tom will be there." Tom, the brother with the smile. Now I had even more reason not to go. I'd just finished a long surgery and I felt sweaty and grubby after hours under the lights. My hair was limp and I had a ring around my head where my surgical cap had left its mark. This is no way to make an impression, I thought, as I scrambled to come up with other reasons to avoid the dinner. But finally I allowed myself to be convinced.

That dinner was the beginning. The next day I found my-self in a car with Tom and four of his Polish employees. I'd learned from his brother that Tom owned a Ukrainian restau-rant in the East Village and most of his employees were Poles. Now I was meeting a group of them and we were heading for a day at the beach. I was the only one who didn't speak Polish and Tom was the only one who spoke English and Polish, but what do you need to say when it's a sunny Sunday and you're on your way to the beach after a long winter?

By the end of that day I knew Tom was someone special. He made me realize what I'd been missing in the men I'd been meeting. He seemed almost "Midwestern" to me in his approach to life—just like me—and I felt instantly at home with him. When I discovered he was a runner and marathoner I enlisted him as my marathon coach. We both had had vague plans to compete in the New York City Marathon, but now they solidified. At best I'd finish the marathon and spend months with Tom preparing for it. At worst I'd spend months with Tom. Either prospect was enticing.

As Tom and I spent more and more time together he inevitably became involved with my animals. He cared for Myriah when my schedule went crazy, he grew to love birds and he helped me out of more than one desperate situation—like Sue the Great.

From the moment Sue arrived at the AMC he was a special case. Not so much because of his malady but because of his look and his personality. Sue was a seven-month-old fawn-colored Great Dane puppy. And Sue was a he. He was big, huge in fact, even for a Great Dane, and he had none of the melancholy of his breed. He was a born clown. His dignified expression, which seemed to deny every ridiculous thing he did, only made him more endearing.

I had been working on a feather picker the night that Sue came in. A feather picker is a bird, usually a large bird like an African gray parrot or an Amazon parrot, although parakeets may be affected as well. A feather picker is easy to spot because it looks like an emperor with no clothes. The feathers are picked off the bodies but the head still has full plumage. The bird has picked off all the feathers he could reach, which includes the plumage all over his body except his head. Their owners usually bring them in thinking they have mites or lice or some skin disease. But when you see a naked bird with a feathered head you know it's a feather picker.

No one is certain what causes a bird to become a feather

picker. Some explanations rely on psychological analysis. This is the "bored bird" school, which holds that a bird becomes a feather picker out of *ennui*. Perhaps the owners aren't playing with him. Perhaps they just had a baby and aren't giving the bird the attention he's accustomed to. Sometimes the owners have just moved and the bird hasn't adjusted to the new environment. Then there's the physical school, which proposes that feather pickers are simply reacting to their molt. Birds usually molt twice a year and sometimes the itch of the old feathers being replaced with new encourages the bird to develop the habit of feather picking.

The solution to feather picking is usually stimulation. Sometimes I recommend the bird be moved to a room that has more activity. Stimulation in the way of toys, music or perhaps more television can sometimes set a bird right. And while you're thinking up ways to stimulate your bird, it's important to break the cycle of picking. We do this by fashioning an Elizabethan collar cut out of X-ray film and fitting it to the bird. Once collared, he can no longer reach his feathers to pick and has to come up with new diversions.

At any rate, I had just finished making the collar for my feather picker when Sue arrived. As he lumbered into the examining room I was struck by the contrast between working on a relatively small and delicate animal like a parrot, where everything, instruments and medications, seemed in miniature, to a Great Dane, where nothing seemed large enough. For example, it was almost impossible to safely get Sue on the examining table so I worked with him on the floor.

His owners had brought him in because that evening he'd begun retching and salivating and his abdomen was distended. Sue had gulped down a large plate of pasta at lunch while the owners were out of the kitchen. This wasn't a difficult feat for him or a new one. He had only to rest his big head on the table and inhale. But he'd never eaten quite so much in the past. Then, later in the day, he'd gone for a romp in the park. It was soon after the run that Sue began to display his symptoms. Concerned, his owners rushed him to the AMC. There were financial as well as emotional considerations: Sue had been bought to be a show dog and his owners were eager to begin working with him. They didn't want anything to stand in the way of future championships.

I immediately figured Sue for a torsion case. He had all the signs. However, he could just be distended versus torsed, so I'd have to confirm my diagnosis with an abdominal X ray so I told the owners that if they wanted to wait a bit, I'd take the X ray and then let them know how I thought we should proceed. When the results were ready I was pleased to have my diagnosis confirmed but sorry to see that Sue had a torsion. It was going to take a bit of work to get him back in fine fettle again.

Unfortunately, stomach torsions are not uncommon. They usually occur in large, deep-chested dogs but they can also afflict smaller breeds. I've even seen basset hounds and poodles who had had a torsion. In a torsion the stomach rotates around on itself, cutting off the circulation and the normal flow of the digestive system. Food is trapped and the stomach becomes distended. As the blood circulation is cut off, parts of the stomach can die. As the stomach swells it presses on the diaphragm and causes heavy, labored breathing. Sometimes the dog retches, sometimes not. But in most cases you can feel the swelling of the stomach and if you tap it with your finger, it sounds taut, like a drum.

Most cases of stomach torsion came in during the evening. People come home from work and they feed their dogs. Then they exercise them. Sometimes they take them running, sometimes they just play roughly, perhaps a vigorous game of fetch. As the dog runs and leaps, his stomach flips over and the trouble starts. Two to six hours after eating they arrive retching and on the verge of shock. A stomach torsion can be a surgical emergency. It's essential to relieve the pressure on the stomach and the surrounding tissues immediately.

I explained the results of the X ray to Sue's owners and

told them all about torsion. Then I explained that I would have to immediately insert a tube into Sue's stomach to get rid of the trapped food. But it was also possible that Sue could later need surgery. The owners left for home and I promised to call them later that evening with news of Sue's condition.

Then I remembered Tom. We were scheduled to have dinner together later. I called and told him about Sue. It looked like it was going to be another late date. He was, as usual, understanding. Thinking of Tom and hoping I wouldn't have to cancel the dinner altogether, I rushed Sue into the prep room and went to work. I put a catheter in his front leg and pumped in fluids and antibiotics. I had to get a tube down into his stomach and then move him into different positions to pass out the food from the stomach through the tube. There were three people working with me, holding Sue down on the table as I stood on a chair to get the tube inserted.

When I pump out a pet's stomach I always feel like I'm looking through the owner's refrigerator in their absence. With torsion cases it's commonly a parade of starches. Pasta and rice are usually main components of the last, offending meal. Most people don't know that foods like pasta and rice absorb water and swell in the dog's stomach and help to cause a torsion by overfilling it. We retrieved an impressive amount of pasta from Sue. After what seemed like hours of pumping we had him empty and stabilized and, tired and hungry. I called his owners to tell them Sue was stabilized and that surgery was indicated. Finally, I called Tom and told him I was on my way.

Tom was by that time used to my version of dinner-table conversation so, as we grabbed a very late bite, I told him about Sue. I was pleased I would be able to give Sue a good prognosis. The only problem was that since he had had a torsion at such a young age, he was likely to have others unless we did a preventive operation. A circumcostal gastropexy is a surgical procedure that takes a bit of the stomach and wraps it around a rib, preventing any future torsions by keeping the stomach sewn into place. Fortunately, Tom found this sort of information interesting and was always willing to listen patiently while I explained in clinical detail the reason for the delay in our dinner.

Sue was doing well the next day and it looked like he would be in the clear for the operation any time in the next few days. I phoned his owners and gave them an update on his condition. I explained that we had temporarily relieved him but that ultimately he would need an operation. If Sue had been an older dog and this was his first torsion, he could probably get by without. He would have to be fed canned food or, if he were fed dried food, it would have to be soaked with water first so it wouldn't expand in his stomach. And he would have to be fed divided feedings: maybe three times a day instead of once. And, of course, he couldn't run or play hard until a few hours after eating. I still recommended the precautions about eating but I told them that without the gastropexy, Sue's chances for the long haul weren't good, as it could potentially recur.

Sue's owners wanted to think about it and said they would call me later in the day. Meanwhile, I had a full roster. There was an elderly Dachshund who had been saved by her owner's attentiveness. She was brought in by an apologetic elderly lady who had noticed a small bump on the dog's belly. The woman was almost certain she was fussing about nothing, but she loved her dog and was worried. . . . I removed the tiny bump, biopsied it and it turned out to be malignant cancer but there was no evidence of any spread to the lymph nodes. The woman's attentiveness had probably saved, or definitely prolonged, her dog's life. As it was, just a few minutes on the examining table and a bit of attention and, if we caught it before it spread, as it seemed at this point, the dog would be good as new. As I watched the lady leave with the dog under her arm—my view was of the back of a small, stooped woman and under one of her arms a brown bundle with an endlessly wagging tail—I thought about how important it is for people to examine their dogs regularly and see to any problem immediately. Unfortunately small problems left unattended are apt to become large ones and heartbroken owners are left with an aching loss and a large bill.

It was immediately after my lucky Dachshund left that I heard from Sue's owners. I had told them the gastropexy would cost anywhere from $600 to $1,000, which surely is expensive, but that we could work out a payment plan. When they called back that afternoon they told me that they didn't want to spend that much money and I had their permission to put Sue to sleep. This was a tricky situation. I couldn't bear to put Sue to sleep but I could certainly understand why someone couldn't afford a possible thousand-dollar vet bill.

I went to my boss and explained the situation. I proposed that, due to the owner's financial situation, we do the operation for cost. It was an unusual case—you rarely see a torsion in such a young dog—and perhaps we could learn something that would prove useful to us in the future if we saw what was going on inside Sue. My boss kindly agreed and I called the people back with the good news. But it seemed that I had misunderstood them. It wasn't that they couldn't afford the cost of the operation; it was that they thought it might be "throwing good money after bad." They had spoken to the breeder and as they'd already spent too much money to buy Sue—he was a fine specimen and highly prized because of his size—they didn't want to sink any more money into him. You could never be sure until a dog reached maturity whether or not he'd be a success in the show ring and these people, on the advice of their breeder, felt that they'd be better off starting over with a new dog than gambling $600 to $1,000 on Sue.

This was another matter entirely. I couldn't convince them Sue was worth the operation, no matter what happened in the show ring. At the same time, I was dismayed by the prospect of putting such a beautiful and delightful dog to sleep.

Toward the end of the conversation, no doubt hearing the

disappointment in my voice and perhaps feeling sheepish about their decision, the owners said I could, if I wanted, fix Sue up and give him away. This wasn't particularly cheering because I couldn't imagine how I would find someone to operate on him and what I would do with him afterward.

After I got off the phone with his owners I went into the wards to visit Sue. As usual, despite the rough treatment he had received at my hands as I removed a few tons of pasta from his belly, he was happy to see me. He banged the cages with his tail, setting up a ringing echo that traveled through the wards. His face, with his black mask, was so expressive he was irresistible. I suspected the aides had given him a treat or two despite the sign "Do Not Feed" tacked to his door. I patted Sue on his massive head and called Tom. I had a plan.

Late that night, after all the regular cases were finished, I performed a gastropexy on Sue. I figured if I kept it quiet, no one would ever know. It wasn't AMC policy to do free surgery on abandoned dogs; therefore I had to do the operation undercover. What I hadn't really figured on was how hard it is to hide a Great Dane.

After the operation Sue really should have had at least twenty-four hours before he was moved. But we didn't have twenty-four hours. We weren't sure the AMC would approve of what we were doing and we didn't want to stick around to find out. So with his catheter still in his leg and a bottle of fluids held aloft, I spirited him out of the AMC. I'd operated on him at 8 P.M. the previous evening and at 6 A.M. Tom drove me to the AMC in his new van to pick up Sue. I knew that things would be quiet then and I'd have a good chance of getting Sue out undetected. As it turned out, carrying a groggy Great Dane and a bottle of fluids cannot be done furtively. But still we tried to be as unobtrusive as possible. Within minutes we were speeding down the FDR Drive and, despite the fact that Sue's catheter leaked, bleeding on his brand-new cream-colored upholstery, Tom was the soul of calm. Praying we wouldn't get stuck in any rush-hour traffic and that somewhere there existed a solution that would get blood out of beige fabric, we got Sue to his temporary destination.

Because I already had Myriah at home as well as two birds and several cats, I knew that Sue wouldn't find a peaceful spot for his recovery at my place. But as luck would have it Tom had just the place for him: Veselka Coffee Shop, Tom's Ukrainian/Polish restaurant in the East Village, a neighborhood that was being dragged into fashionability by the escalating rents everywhere else in the city. The Veselka had a basement where even a convalescent Great Dane would be comfortable. The fact that Tom was willing to risk his livelihood for the sake of a strange dog made me realize all over again how special he was. Sue was calm during the journey, but when we got to Ninth Street and Second Avenue, he suddenly made a bolt for freedom. Tom and I were trying to maneuver him from the backseat when he jumped free and headed for Second Avenue. You'll see many things on the Lower East Side. People with hair every color of the rainbow. A man who walks around with a giant stuffed eagle. Another who roller skates in a dress holding a sort of magic wand. But I bet Sue was the first postop Great Dane on the scene. He dashed to the corner with his catheter trailing behind him, bandages flapping about his middle and he drew hardly a stare.

When we finally collared Sue and got him down to the basement of the Veselka we could hardly believe it was only 8 A.M. It seemed we had been up and about for days. But Sue was finally safe, barricaded into the corner with his fluid bottle hung on a convenient pipe. It was time for me to get to work so I left Tom with instructions on how to adjust Sue's catheter.

Sue's recovery was not uneventful. Tom and I spoke on the phone countless times that day. The catheter seemed to be clogged. The catheter seemed to be flowing too fast. But Tom didn't trouble me with the incidental problems. For example, the fact that Sue got very rambunctious and pulled down a shelf of dishes. That Sue got bored and chewed clear through his catheter and sat happily as the fluids dribbled across the floor. That the Ukrainian pastry chef arrived in the afternoon and descended into the basement only to ricochet back up to the dining room in record time hollering about a "monster" in the basement. All this was made more confusing because the pastry chef doesn't speak English. But Tom held the fort, and when I got there after a full day at the AMC, Sue was doing as well as could be expected. The Veselka was in chaos but Sue was on the mend. It was obvious he needed a new home and fast.

The second night of Sue's recovery, fearing for Tom's restaurant, we moved Sue to his nearby apartment. We barricaded Tom's cats into various rooms and let Sue lumber about. He seemed so docile, so endearing, so harmless. Thus lulled, we let one of the cats into the living room. Sue regarded the cat with interest. The cat, who was used to Myriah's visits, was unconcerned. But suddenly Sue decided to make a rush for her. An instant before he lunged, I saw what was happening. I made a grab for Sue while Tom went for the cat. Well, even in his weakened state, I couldn't hang on to Sue and so, with Tom and me in pursuit, he chased the cat into the bedroom, where she sat on the highest bookshelf, hissing and complaining. Was the cat hurt? We couldn't tell without examining her and so, while I held Sue as best I could, Tom tried to rescue the very unwilling cat. When he at last managed to get high enough to grab her, she simultaneously bit him and urinated on him. Poor Tom. Dating a vet surely has its disadvantages. But it was his kindness and steely calm in just such situations that were convincing me he was someone I wanted to be in my life always. But we still had to find another solution to Sue.

The astonishingly effective grapevine at the AMC was given word that a home was needed for a beautiful Great Dane puppy. It seemed that within hours I had the name of a family in New Jersey. If Sue, who was back in the Veselka basement, could get through one more day without tearing down the entire establishment, all would be well. We took extra precautions. We leashed Sue to one wall so he couldn't escape and terrify the help. We set up a heat lamp to keep Sue warm. And we moved every item that Sue could knock down, chew or otherwise destroy out of harm's way.

On the evening of the third day of Sue's recovery we loaded him into the van (after covering the seats with a sheet) and set off for New Jersey. Sue was an interested passenger throughout the ride and I kept hoping he wasn't memorizing landmarks so that he could find his way back to Veselka and the bits of cheese danish the pastry chef had begun tossing him in an effort to stay on his good side. The new family lived in a beautiful house with a giant yard in a countrified suburb about two hours from Manhattan. When we pulled into the driveway they were lined up by the front door like a Norman Rockwell illustration. When the door to the van slid open, Sue bounded across the lawn and onto the porch as if returning home at last. The two children were thrilled to have a dog, once they got over the fact that the dog was so much bigger than they were. I was delighted to have found such a good situation for Sue and he seemed to share my enthusiasm. Tom and I were invited in for a cup of coffee and we told the family what Sue's operation had been for and how to care for him. I glossed over his origins and then I bent down to hug Sue good-bye. As I put my arms around his powerful neck he wagged his giant tail, sending an ashtray and a small vase of flowers sailing off the coffee table and onto the stone hearth. I winked at Tom, who returned my grin. We both knew the family was going to have to Sue-proof their house.

Recently I heard from Sue's new family. He's fully recovered and they can't imagine life without him. His name is Hamlet now and his owners are convinced that when he's fully grown, he'll become more graceful.

Oh yes, and Tom's cat bites have healed, most of the blood came out of the van's upholstery and the Ukrainian pastry chef, whose first English words were "big dog," now laughs about the monster Sue.

HESITATION

The sun was streaming in my window and that's what woke me. I was scheduled for a double shift that day. I probably wouldn't get off work until near midnight. I wouldn't see Tom till the next day or maybe the day after if our schedules got crazy. There was nothing unusual about that morning or the day ahead of me except the way I felt. For the first time since beginning work as a vet I was unhappy. But my state of mind was really a paradox: on the one hand I was defeated. My work had become routine, routine but endlessly demanding. But my personal life was more full and happy than it had ever been before. I spent every free minute with Tom and I hated to leave him. Each long hour at the AMC was one stolen from Tom, or really from me, because it seemed I was only really me when I was with Tom.

I sat on the edge of my bed watching Myriah as she begged for breakfast. There had been so many mornings when I'd leaped out of bed, eager to get to the AMC and check on my cases. How could all that pleasure and excitement have vanished? I still cared about the animals; what seemed hollow to me was the vision of my career, the vision that had kept me going through vet school, my first job, my internship and the beginning of my residency. I no longer wanted to be the best vet in the world. I wanted to be happy.

So this is how it happens, I thought, as I finally went to the kitchen and poured kibble into Myriah's metal bowl. You work and struggle and then you fall in love and nothing else matters. Considered in that light, my feelings made me ashamed. I saw all the farmers in Ohio who'd watched with skepticism as I'd palpated their cows and stuck their pigs. They knew all along.

Myriah found me standing by the window in the sunshine. With her precise sense of order and time, she seemed dismayed to see me staring at traffic as the minutes ticked by. She was always ready for the next event. Only food completely diverted her, I thought, with affection as I considered for the thousandth time how amazing it was that she could eat so fast and with such total concentration. Life is easy for animals because of their simple inclinations: one thing at a time, each thing in its proper order. A walk, a meal, a rest, a ride, another walk, another meal, another nap and time for bed everyone. No splitting yourself between work and love. No hesitation. Each day a pin to be knocked down in its time.

I knew I should be dressing. If I didn't leave in ten minutes I'd be late. But instead of heading for my closet I picked up the phone.

"Tom, let's have breakfast. Are you free?"

"But Sally, I thought you had to work. Aren't you on a double today?"

"Do you have another breakfast date?" I laughed.

"Okay. Come on over. We just pulled some apple cinnamon muffins out of the oven."

I rushed to get dressed, suddenly filled with all the energy and enthusiasm that had deserted me when faced with the prospect of work. As I walked the busy morning streets to Veselka I knew what I had to do. I decided to quit the AMC. I'd already had more training than the vast majority of vets. I'd completed my internship, more than I'd ever hoped to accomplish five years ago. What was the point of continuing my residency? If I left now I could have breakfast with Tom all the time. I could get a regular job as a vet somewhere in the city. I'd make a real salary and for the first time in years would have money to spend. I'd buy some nice clothes. Tom and I could go to the theater. Maybe go on real vacations. No more Tom sitting for an hour in the AMC lobby as one un-expected thing after another delayed me. No more weekends lost to emergency duty. No more last-minute canceled plans. Best of all would be ordinary mornings just like this that I could spend with Tom.

I made my way along Second Avenue in a state of joy. Why had it taken me so long to realize what I really wanted? When

I'd called the AMC to tell them I wouldn't be in, it was as if an enormous weight had slipped from me. I was free. I could chart my course and I would. If it felt that good simply to skip a day of work wasn't that a sign?

Tom was shocked by my decision. As the morning crowd of punk types mixed with regular uptown business people ebbed and flowed around us and the delicious smells of bacon, eggs, and coffee drifted in invisible clouds through the restaurant, I explained my plan.

"But what about your residency?" Tom wanted to know.

"I don't need my residency. I need to live like a normal person, that's what I need."

Tom was dubious. His lack of enthusiasm stunned me. He listened carefully but he didn't seem to pick up on the great happiness I'd found for myself. Didn't he want to spend more time with me? I couldn't bring myself to ask the question but it certainly dulled my pleasure.

The only argument Tom had for my staying at the AMC was based on what he knew of the old me—the me before I fell in love with him—the me that had wanted to be the very best vet in the world and to pour myself into nothing but work. He knew how I'd loved the AMC. How I'd rush to work. How I'd talk about my cases endlessly. How engrossed I was in veterinary medicine. How could I expect him to understand the new me in the course of a breakfast; I hardly understood myself.

The decision was mine and I'd made it. I knew that shortly Tom would realize it was the best for me, for us. Now I had to tell the AMC. I'd go right up there after breakfast and get it over with and then Tom and I would have the rest of the day, no, we'd have weeks, months. In fact, I'd take some time off before I began a new job and we'd work our time around his restaurant responsibilities. It would be heaven.

Sitting in the small plain office with my boss at the AMC, I was in a tumult. Everything was oddly quiet, or maybe it was just that I wasn't in a rush. I'd never moved slowly in that building before. Already I was beginning to peel myself away, I thought, and a good thing too. For too long I'd seen the world from one perspective. Now I'd begin to really live.

It was the idea of broadening and improving myself, of finally arriving at a sane balance, that sustained me. Because if I paused for too long in my explanation, I began to feel like an ungrateful child. Despite my success, I'd spent all my veterinary education feeling like a bit of an underdog. I suppose because it had been so hard to get that volunteer job, so hard to get into school, so hard to find my way. It was all a gift and here I was refusing it. But I couldn't allow myself to be undermined by a vague guilt, a feeling that was, after all, a figment of my imagination. I'd done my best. I'd done well and it was time for a change.

My boss was skeptical. He didn't believe me. First Tom and now him. It was enormously frustrating to undergo a sea change that no one else could appreciate or even believe. He wouldn't accept my resignation. He'd give me a leave of absence for one week. Then I could decide. I could decide right now, I thought, but I'll give him a week. It would make for a more graceful exit.

That week of early summer, the week that was to be an idyllic transition to my new life of freedom, turned out to be the week that never was. One minute it was Monday morning, the next was Sunday night. Tom and I did get to breakfast together a few times. We had a couple of dinners on schedule. But the leisurely trips to the beach, the romantic afternoons, the endless summer evenings—they never happened. We'd planned to do a lot of running together but on Tuesday I pulled a muscle in my leg. So much for a week of dedicated training. And there were so many interruptions, mainly unexpected things that happened at Veselka. I'd been unaware of the strange rhythms of the restaurant because I'd always been at work. But there seemed to be a crisis a day: a dishwasher out, a waitress wanting to switch schedules because she had an audition, a late delivery. I'd known that Tom would be working but somehow in my vision of the week things had been different.

But the real problem that week wasn't how I filled my days, it was the echo of how I used to fill my days. I'd find myself with an hour or two to kill and I couldn't settle on what to do. Go to a museum? I'd never had time before. How about exploring SoHo? Or maybe trying one of the sales I'd seen advertised in the paper? More often then not I'd find myself doing meaningless chores in a bustle of indecision.

Toward the end of the week Tom and I were driving south on the FDR Drive. He pointed out a huge sailboat that was fighting the current upriver. But we were at Sixty-second Street and I was looking the other way, toward the AMC. I would have been on phone duty at that hour. I wondered how my cases were doing. The place looked so dirty from the outside. And that's where I was—on the outside. I was a civilian now. Tom glanced from the sailboat to see what had my attention. Our eyes met and we smiled at one another but said nothing.

Sunday was a beautiful day. My first free Sunday, I thought, as Tom and I planned a morning trip to the beach. It was early in the season, early in the day, and the crowds wouldn't be bad. I could afford to really relax. Next week or maybe the week after, I'd begin to look for a job in the city. I could take a part-time job at the ASPCA any time I wanted. And if I didn't want something permanent, there were always practices that were delighted to have a regular substitute, especially one with my AMC experience. A job would be no problem.

The beach was nearly deserted at that early hour. Still we had to take our time to pick the very best spot. Far from any radios. Just near enough to the surf. Close enough to feel the breath of the spray but not so close that we'd be in a line of traffic. The feeling of the sun hitting my skin was delicious. Resting my head on my arm, I watched the tiny blond hairs on my arm tremble and felt my world was very perfect and contained. Eventually Tom goaded me into a swim but the water was still too cold to really enjoy. When we were toweling ourselves back on our blanket, panting and blowing and shaking our wet heads like grounded seals, Tom turned to me with a smile and said, "Have you decided what to do, Sally?"

"About what?"

"About the AMC."

We hadn't really discussed it all week. Of course we hadn't. There wasn't really anything to discuss. But looking at Tom at that moment with his wet hair and his strong face I knew why there'd been nothing to discuss. I was still the old me. The old me plus Tom. This week hadn't been what I'd expected. I couldn't live Myriah's simple life, one thing at a time. The question of how to balance my life was answered. It wasn't a matter of carving up the day into the appropriate pieces; it was a matter of having the right person in my life, someone who perhaps knew me better than I knew myself.

"Well, I suppose I'll stop by tomorrow. I guess my leave is up."

Tom leaned over and kissed me on the forehead. He didn't say anything. It was as if he'd known all along.

DOLLY DOES THE JOB

After a year my internship at the AMC was over but I was accepted to continue as a medical resident, specializing in gastroenterology. As a resident I had more responsibility in our medical service and I was also in charge of all the endoscopy. Endoscopy is the procedure of passing a flexible tube down the esophagus and into the stomach. It's an extremely useful procedure that allows you to inspect for ulcers and tumors and also to remove foreign bodies. Despite my slightly higher status, I still occasionally saw clients who didn't believe I was a doctor. Sometimes because I was a woman or sometimes because I looked too young, they would be doubtful of my capabilities. I could always spot this kind of person because they would scrutinize my nameplate and often ask if I was in fact a full-fledged doctor. Despite the fact that I'd now had almost three years more training than the average vet, they would sometimes still be skeptical. I remember one disheveled fellow who brought a cocker spaniel puppy in to me to be vaccinated. He took one disgusted look at me and said, "I was expecting a doctor who shaves." Undaunted, I smiled and replied, "I was expecting a client who shaves."

As I felt more and more at home at the AMC as a resident I began to understand the system and anticipate the inevitable problems I would encounter. Given the size of the staff and the clientele at the AMC, it was amazing that there weren't more wrinkles, bulges and backups in the flow of the daily routines.

One of the rivalries that kept everyone on his toes was that between the medical staff and the surgical staff. The medical staff, of which I was a member, was responsible to a client from the moment they came in the door with a pet. We'd examine the animal, come up with a diagnosis and treatment and, with luck, send the animal home healthy. We thought of ourselves as the primary caretakers and we also were the link between the AMC and the clients. In our most impatient and conceited moments we saw the surgeons as mere technicians. And sometimes the surgeons saw us as people who simply wanted to dump difficult cases on them to solve. They no doubt felt that whenever we couldn't find what was wrong with an animal, we sent it to surgery. The truth lay somewhere in between.

When a case we were working on required a surgical procedure in the course of treatment, we'd "turf to surge," or turn the case over to the surgical staff. In most cases we'd schedule a surgery and things would go smoothly, but because of the traditional rivalry between the two staffs sometimes a surgeon would "ding" or cancel a surgery you had requested. The surgeon always had a good reason for this; in many cases he would feel that he was doing a "live postmortem," meaning that the case was going to die anyhow so the procedure you had scheduled was a waste of time and money. And no surgeon wants to operate if he doesn't think the procedure will be a success. Or sometimes the surgeon would decide that a few more diagnostic tests were in order before the animal was to be operated on. But sometimes there was no other way to determine what, exactly, was wrong with an animal without going in and looking and so you'd have to argue your case until you convinced the surgical staff you were right. I think in the long run the sense the medical and surgical people had of being in two different camps worked to everyone's benefit as a sort of informal system of checks and balances, though no one would have liked to admit it.

A more persistent problem at the AMC was the low blood supply. We rarely had as big a blood supply as we could have wished. Sometimes when an animal needed a transfusion we had to struggle to get our hands on the required amount of blood. One solution to this was the donor dogs. We often had dogs kept in a pen in the wards who were used as blood donors. Every few weeks we'd take some blood from each dog and replenish our supply. Sometimes vets would bring in their own dogs to donate blood at times when blood was in demand. Sometimes we'd use drop-off dogs that people had abandoned on our doorstep. If they were sick we cured them and used them for a short time as donors while we found a home for them. It was really quite a fair arrangement and both the dog and the AMC benefitted.

One dilemma that caused the staff at the AMC headaches was the cost of our services. There was no doubt about it, our costs were high. Not unreasonably high, but higher than some of the local vets. Given the sophistication of our equipment and the training of our specialists, it isn't surprising that we cost more. But still, there were always some clients who were shocked, dismayed or just plain angry when their bill came.

We tried to avoid these problems by telling a client early on what we thought a given treatment would cost. It's often difficult to tell in advance exactly what a pet's bill will be but I always made a point of being as specific as possible. And I also tried to be understanding about people's financial difficulties.

There was one particularly memorable incident involving the costs of care at the AMC. It began somewhere in a vet's office in New Jersey. A French bulldog named Dolly had been brought to see this vet because she was becoming increasingly sick. She was vomiting and had a severe case of diarrhea. The New Jersey vet thought she was suffering from kidney failure and treated her accordingly, but every time he took her off the intravenous fluids, her kidney tests elevated again. Dolly kept failing and her owners were heartbroken. The two ladies who owned Dolly bred pugs and French bulldogs. Dolly, though she wasn't a show prospect, was a particular favorite. And Dolly was a young dog—about four years old and very young to have kidney failure. So when the New Jersey vet recommended that they put Dolly to sleep, they just couldn't bring themselves to do it. They told him they wanted to take her to New York to the AMC and get a second opinion.

It was at this point that the pressure to get rid of Dolly began. First with the vet, who just couldn't believe that a dog with kidney failure was worth saving. Then with the ladies' breeder friends. "Why not just put the poor dear to sleep?" they'd all say. "You'll be putting her out of her misery and besides it could cost a fortune to keep testing her and treating her and what for? What good can come of it?"

But the ladies loved Dolly and so they prevailed and brought her to the AMC. The first vet who saw her took a history, examined her, reviewed the blood work from the referring vet, and immediately diagnosed her as an Addisonian. She was suffering from Addison's disease, a failure of the adrenal glands to produce enough cortisone for the body. This disease commonly mimics kidney failure and is commonly mistaken as such, which is what the New Jersey vet had done.

I took over Dolly's case shortly after she was admitted to

the hospital. I enjoyed meeting the two delightful women who owned her and I enjoyed meeting Dolly herself, who had a shiny black and white coat and the lolling tongue typical of the French bulldog. She was spirited and intelligent and, if she never took a ribbon in a show, she was still a wonderful specimen. I could quickly see how these women couldn't bear to lose her.

An Addisonian, fortunately, can be treated with medication and can live a full life. But stabilizing her in the hospital is expensive. I made a long phone call to the ladies in New Jersey to tell them what had to be done to cure Dolly, who was still at the AMC undergoing tests, and what it would cost. The total cost could be near $1,000. There wasn't a moment's hesitation. They wanted Dolly well. They told me that all their friends thought they were crazy and were wasting their money and that they'd do much better to forget Dolly and concentrate on their other dogs but they'd have none of it.

Over the period of Dolly's treatment I got to know the ladies well. And once Dolly went home I kept in touch with her progress with frequent phone conversations. Within a short period of time at home, Dolly was doing beautifully. She was so intelligent and sweet that if the ladies ever forgot to give Dolly her daily medication, Dolly would stand by the medicine cabinet and bark to remind them. This struck me as particularly unusual as so many pets hate to take medication and I'm often giving advice on how to disguise pills by hiding them in a meatball or peanut butter or coating them with butter so they'll slide down the throat. The ladies were still taking some criticisms from their friends about the cost of Dolly's medical care but now that she was her lively and spirited self, these comments were readily dismissed by Dolly's owners.

Then one day the ladies had a party at their house near the shore in New Jersey. There'd been quite a crowd—lots of dog people and local friends and everyone had had a lovely time. When the last car had pulled away the ladies retreated to their rooms exhausted. They were awakened at two in the morning by Dolly's low growl. Both women waited silently in their rooms. A few minutes passed and they both heard someone knock softly at the door. It must be one of their guests who had forgotten something, they thought as they met in the hall and moved toward the door. But as they padded across the kitchen, they heard someone trying to jimmy the lock. Frozen in terror, they watched as the doorknob rattled. All of this happened in just a few seconds and Dolly was at their sides, quietly waiting, it seemed, for their reaction so that she'd know how to approach this problem. When it became clear they were frightened, Dolly began to bark and growl ferociously. Now Dolly, like the average French bulldog, weighed only about twenty pounds and had been originally bred to hunt mice. But she was barking with the savagery of a dog ten times her size. Each bark lifted the entire front half of her body off the floor and she resembled a black and white wind-up toy as she made her progress across the floor.

The ladies stood pressed against the wall in fear, watching Dolly, watching the door. Their car was in the driveway and the fact that the intruder could see it frightened them even more. If he knew someone was at home and still was trying to break in, it didn't bode well for them. But when Dolly first began to bark, the door knob stopped moving. And as she continued her assault, there was only silence outside. Then, after what must have seemed like hours, the ladies saw a shadowy figure race across their lawn and over their fence. Dolly was at last silent. She sat on the kitchen floor, panting furiously and looking from face to face as if to ask why everyone didn't just go back to bed and forget this nonsense as there was no longer anyone at the door.

The police were called, the neighborhood was searched, but no one was ever found. The ladies were just as glad, they told me. I heard the whole story from them the day they came in with Dolly to pose for photo. They wanted a picture of me holding Dolly. It would be published in the French bulldog magazine—*Frenchie Bullytin*—along with a story of how the cost of curing Dolly had been small indeed given the return she had made. They were convinced that Dolly had saved their lives, and who's to say she hadn't?

A NEW BEGINNING

I would be in a beautiful white gown. Everyone would say afterward that it was the most extraordinary dress they'd ever seen. The ceremony would be in a small chapel in the woods near Mentor. All my friends and family would be there. Lorraine, Lesley, Skid . . . and my new friends from the AMC would come to Ohio for the event. Of course it would be in the summer so everything could be outdoors and I'd be tan and radiant. When we entered the chapel, Myriah would proceed us, carrying a basket filled with flowers in her mouth. And I'd stand in the back watching her tail sway gently as she moved with great dignity to the altar. Then the bridesmaids and finally me on my father's arm. And of course Tom would be waiting for me, Myriah sitting next to him, to begin our life together.

Well, it didn't quite work out like that. The chapel was too small to hold everyone I wanted to invite. And I never convinced anyone, myself included, to be honest, that Myriah would bring off the event without a hitch. She waited at home. But my friends and family were all there, it was in August, the dress was beautiful and Tom was waiting for me at the altar.

Now the AMC is behind me. I'm working at a practice on the East Side of Manhattan and living in the East Village. My schedule is still frantic. Tom has his own pressures. The restaurant business is one of long hours and frequent crises. We eat most of our meals at the Veselka. Our apartment in the East Village does not have a white picket fence. But my dream has come true.